Chair Yoga for Seniors Over 60

A Simple Guide to Regain Muscle Flexibility and Balance in the Comfort of your own Home, with an Easy Exercise Routine

Table of Contents

Sommario

Introduction 6
   What Is Chair Yoga, and What Are the Benefits of Practicing It? 6

Chapter1: Breathing Techniques & Meditation (Pranayama) 9
   The Pranayama Mudras 11
   Ideal Position for Pranayama 16

Chapter 2: Warm-up 23
   Warm-Ups You Can Do in a Chair 23
   Neck Movements 25
   Shoulder Exercise 28
   Exercises for Arms and Elbows 28
   Exercises for the Back and Abdominal Area 29
   Exercises for the Legs 29
   Ankle and Foot Exercises 30
   Warm-up Exercises for Arms and Back 30
   Trunk Warm-up Exercises 31
   Injuries That Can Occur Due to a Bad Warm-up 31
   Muscle Cramps 31

Chapter 3: Beginners Program 33
   Neck Wheels 33
   Shoulder Circles 35
   Lateral Stretch From Chair 35
   Lateral Stretch Exercise Holding Onto the Chair 36
   Twists in a Chair 36
   Activating the Torso 36
   Expanding the Chest 37

Hands Up 37

Head Up 37

Pigeon Pose 38

Lunge Variation 39

Sitting With Hands on Chest 39

Cactus Arms 40

Healing Plantar Fasciitis 40

Healing Foot Pain 41

Hamstring Stretch 41

Cat and Cow 42

Hand Chest 43

Chapter 4: Intermediate Program 44

Mountain Chair Pose 44

Expanding Chest 45

Torso Circles 45

Floating on the Chair 46

Knees and Head Down 46

Camel Pose 47

Table Pose and Knee-to-Nose Flow Pose 47

Tied Angle Pose 48

Squat Against the Wall in a Standing Position 48

Back-to-Back Chair Pose 49

The Elevator 49

Constructive Rest 49

Garland Pose 54

Hugs, Twists, and Turns 55

Half Easy Pose and Half Forward Bend Pose 55

Broken Wings Pose 56

Pose With Folding Blanket Blocks 56

Chapter 5: Advanced Program 58

Mountain Chair 58
Neck Bends 58
Turning the Neck 59
Cat Pose 60
Cobra Pose 60
Chair Twist 61
Volcano Pose 61
Standing Rolling Down 62
Child's Table Pose 63
Needle Pose 63
Cobra Dance Pose 64
Fish Pose 65
Puppy Pose with Wall Pose 65
Circle of Joy Pose 66
Square Breathing 66
Downward Facing Dog Pose 67
Warrior Chair Pose 68
Corpse Pose 69

Chapter 6: Friendly Poses 71
Connecting in Awareness 71
Giving Love to Shoulders and Arms 71
Mountain Pose Standing With Raised Hands 72
Hand Stretch on the Chair Top 72
Seated Cactus 72
Kundalini Circle 72
Twists Sitting on a Chair 73
To Open your Back 74
Raising Hands 75
The Seated Cobra 75
Pigeon on the Chair 75

Upward Facing Dog 76
Table Pose Raised to Gain Stability 76
High Lunge Pose 77
Triangle Pose 78
Reverse Warrior Pose 79
Chair Boat 80
Pose Upward Straddling 81
Wind Release Pose 81
Downward-Facing Dog in a Chair With Knees Bent 82
Standing Squat Pose 82
Forward Fold with Two Chairs 83
Half Seated Pose 84
Leg Lift Pose 84
Stretched Side Angle 85

Conclusion 87

Yoga Improves Balance and Coordination 87
Your Mind and Body Become Better Connected 87
Your Circulation Improves 87
Your Posture Improves 88
Lower Your Stress and Anxiety Levels 88

☐ THERE IS A SURPRISE FOR YOU ☐

☐ **A GIFT FOR YOU** ☐

☐ **SCAN NOW** ☐

What Will You Receive by Clicking?
☐ An Easy and Comprehensive Guide
☐♀☐ Practical Tips and Techniques
☐ An Holistic Approach

...And a your rating is appreciated. Thank you!!
https://www.amazon.com/review/create-review?&ASIN=B0C6FMWXFQ

Adrienne Fox
StayHealthy

misterbondwriter@gmail.com

Introduction

What Is Chair Yoga, and What Are the Benefits of Practicing It?

Chair Yoga for Seniors *Over 60* allows you to expand your range of possibilities with new movements that are perfectly usable at an old age.

In addition, *Chair Yoga for Seniors Over 60* also allows you to perform traditional yoga movements more comfortably in your home or in any open space, as well as providing you with a greater sense of security without having to worry about untimely falls.

It is very wise to keep in mind the following tips for seniors doing yoga in a chair:

- It is important to check that the chair is in the optimal sitting position, as it may have ill-fitting parts that prevent proper yoga practice.

- Make sure there are no objects around, such as wires, clothing, or even toys, that could become an obstacle and cause a lot of damage if dropped.

- Having enough space in the house to practice yoga is recommended.

- A chair should be placed on a non-slip surface, such as a mat or a stretchy reel, similar to those used for exercising at home; it can also be placed on the grass.

- When practicing yoga, keep your back straight at a 90-degree angle and keep your feet flat on the floor.

From the age of 70, with the onset of joint problems and other diseases, older people have entered a sedentary stage, so it is especially recommendable that these people practice yoga.

Over the years, this practice has spread throughout the world, and many schools or professionals in this field are dedicated to incorporating the routine of yoga exercises for older adults into their programs.

6 out of 10 people who practice yoga are females, and the practice is more frequent among women due to anatomical reasons, which gives them a relative advantage over men. They can easily perform postures that require a certain degree of flexibility. The practice of yoga also offers the following advantages:

- It reduces symptoms of depression and anxiety in older adults.
- It favors the conciliation of sleep, helping to solve the problem of insomnia you may suffer.
- It is a discipline that has a significant impact on the mood of people since doing yoga increases serotonin levels, which notably improves older adults suffering from depression and anxiety.
- The classes are directly related to memory improvement, a very beneficial aspect for seniors with dementia.

This book is not exclusively for seniors over the age of 60. It is made for anyone who cannot practice traditional yoga and wishes to enjoy its benefits, such as someone who has had surgery and cannot move much, obese people, or those who have neurological conditions that prevent them from doing a full exercise class but can be adapted with the support of the chair.

Chair yoga involves lighter exercises than the traditional practice but is just as effective. It is ideal for those who want to get back to exercise but have been inactive for a long time. It can also be used by those who are confined to a wheelchair due to an accident or condition.

For example, Mrs. Steward, who is 67 years old and lives alone in a duplex apartment, had long felt that climbing the stairs had become an ordeal for her. After she learned about chair yoga, she tried it for the first time and discovered from the very first day how her body became more energetic and gradually became more elastic. Today, she climbs stairs easily, as if she had rejuvenated a few years, not to mention when she has to bend down or change position.

Although, as I mentioned before, this book is not just for seniors. David, who has spina bifida, had a lot of trouble getting around. His mother has always tried to help him move, and when he discovered chair yoga, he began to do the stretches with her help to move his feet, arms, neck, and back, and he has noticed progress; he looks better and more balanced, and this book serves as a guide to help him exercise his body.

In old age, when the body no longer responds as it once did and the mind begins to cloud, dementia does not prevent the practice of chair yoga. Sarah helps her 89-year-old mother with dementia; she sits her down every day before grooming her and they exercise. She helps her stretch her arms and places her in the correct postures according to the asana. Sarah adjusts her mother's body nicely, and she seems to follow directions, tensing when appropriate and relaxing when necessary.

As I said at the beginning, yoga is for everyone, and if people want to enjoy their children growing up, their parents, their grandchildren, and as many things as possible without being limited by age or pain, what better than to do yoga in a chair?

Chapter1: Breathing Techniques & Meditation (Pranayama)

In ancient Hindu Sanskrit, *prana* means energy or life force (breath), and *ayama* means to control or regulation. Thus, prana and ayama (pranayama) create breath control. This is what I intend for you to learn in this first chapter.

As mentioned in the Atharva Veda, an ancient Indian religious text dating from 1000 to 900 B.C., people have been practicing pranayama breathing techniques as a yogic breathing exercise for thousands of years.

Practitioners of these breathing techniques have gained countless benefits over the past three millennia. Today, yoga classes often include pranayama (yogic breathing) as part of the practice, but it can be done independently. These techniques certainly apply to the type of yoga we will study.

How These Techniques Work

Pranayama and deep breathing yoga address the one essential point that the human body can automatically control: the breath.

When people tap into the power of the breath through yogic breathing, they create a connection between body and mind. Those who do so can fundamentally change how they think, feel, and act.

The goal of pranayama is to help you achieve and maintain a consistent breathing pattern as you do the *asanas*, the Sanskrit word for yoga postures. Each inhalation should be done deeply and slowly. When you breathe in this way, the vagus nerve is put into action. The vagus nerve runs from the brain to the abdomen. It is responsible for triggering the relaxation response and deactivating our fight or flight reflex, which often occurs under stress.

In short, calming the body calms the mind, and it all starts with deep breathing exercises.

How the Technique Works in Yoga

Yoga is very focused on breathing. Many yoga teachers make this activity the center of their teaching style. You can't do yoga without paying special attention to breathing patterns, which can be developed and shaped by applying pranayama techniques in *hatha* or flow yoga classes.

Advantages of Pranayama

The benefits of this type of exercise are that you can improve sleep and reduce muscle tension, allowing you to clear your mind and stay focused. Here are some specific benefits you can get from practicing pranayama:

- It improves your sleep; you will sleep more and with quality.
- Your attention and concentration improve.
- Your heart health and breathing can be better.
- You will have better digestion and a more regulated metabolism.
- You will have better cognitive performance.
- Anxiety and stress are reduced.
- You have a better mood.
- Your immune system improves.
- Your vital energy increases.

The Complexity of Learning

It is not difficult at all. Pranayama techniques are simple to learn.

While certain types of pranayama breathing may take longer and are more advanced, beginners can start with simple techniques and add them to their daily routine when doing chair exercises.

There are different variations of this deep breathing technique, such as:

- Bhastrika pranayama (Bellows breathing)
- Bhramari pranayama
- Dirga pranayama
- Kapalabhati pranayama (Bright Skull Breathing)

- Alternate nasal breathing
- Simhasana pranayama
- Ujjayi pranayama (known as victorious breathing or oceanic breathing, or ujjayi breathing)

Those beginning in pranayama or chair yoga should consider these last two exercises because they are among the elemental ones in deep breathing.

The Pranayama Mudras

What is Mudra

Mudra is a Sanskrit word, that signifies "Seal," "Gesture," or "Sign" in the official Indian language.

Mudras are symbolic hand and finger movements, to enhance the movement of energy through the body during meditation. Used in conjunction with breathing exercises, they can increase the flow of prana throughout the body, activating the various body areas involved in breathing.

Since the Mudra makes a direct link with the nerves, it also makes a subtle connection with the brain's instinctive patterns, which affects these regions' automatic reactions. When internal energy is adjusted and redirected, changes occur in the tendons, glands, and sensory organs.

The correct position of the hands is extremely important in meditation. Each mudra stimulates different parts of our brain helping us to conduct energy to a certain area of our body. In addition, it is related to the five natural elements and each finger represents a point of connection with an element and the energy connected to it. By positioning our fingers in a certain way, we can control the amount of elemental energy flowing within us.

Energies associated with each site of the hand:
- Thumb: sun, energy, fire.
- Index: air, energy in motion.
- Medium: space, expansion, openness.
- Ring finger: earth, solidity, rootedness.
- Little finger: water, liquids, mobility.

Benefits that can be gained from practicing Prana Mudra:
- Improves the regulating power of the mind
- Decreases nervousness and improves self-confidence.
- Allows you to counteract chronic fatigue, tiredness and lack of patience
- It helps to manage emotions such as anger, fear, mental tension, but also joy, happiness and desire
- Improves attention and presence of mind
- Boosts the immune system
- Improves the digestive system
- Allows you to solve vision problems, such as burning, dry eyes, weak vision and cataracts

The most common mudras and their meaning

Anjali Mudra

The most famous one, associated with namaste

How to do it: join the palms and fingers of the hands, in a prayer position, leaving a very small space between the two palms without stiffening the hands excessively, so that the energy flows. Each finger must adhere perfectly to the finger of the opposite hand and look upwards. The hands are at chest level, in front of the heart.

Meaning: in yoga it is a greeting position, which also favors the balance of energies. It helps to unite and balance the two sides of the body and connect the two hemispheres of the brain.

Benefits: this position is perfect for deep relaxation, to clarify thoughts and to balance our energies, centering us before starting our meditation.

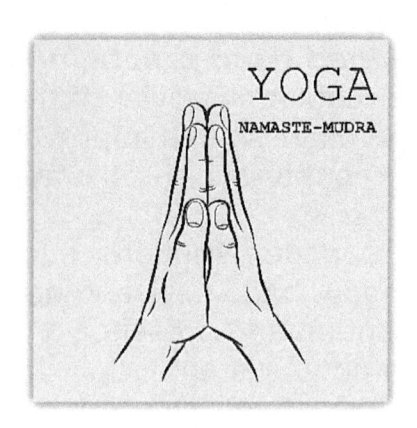

Dhyana Mudra

How to do it: place the back of your left hand on the palm of your right hand and arch your hands slightly as if to form a bowl. You can rest your left thumb on top of your right. The fingers and hands are not tense, but remain relaxed. The more concave the hands, the more energy can flow. The hands rest on the lap, at the height of the second chakra. The right hand symbolizes enlightenment, while the left is the illusory character of existence.

Meaning: This mudra is known as the seal of meditation. The semicircle formed by the hands symbolizes the emptiness to be filled with a new awareness, a gesture of absolute balance.

Benefits: this position deeply calms the mind, frees from anxiety and stress and helps to reach a deep stillness more easily. It also helps eliminate the ego and foster connection with our inner self.

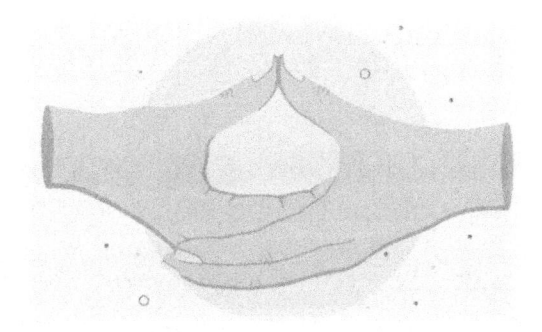

Gyan Mudra

How to do it: the index finger touches the thumb lightly and the other fingers remain relaxed, never tense. It seems that this was the Buddha's favorite mudra during his meditations, and it is also the most widely used nowadays.

Meaning: expresses knowledge, where the index finger characterizes awareness and its union, while the thumb represents the wisdom and expansion of the ego.

What benefits it brings: This posture is used to stimulate creativity and concentration, which also remain at the end of the meditation session.

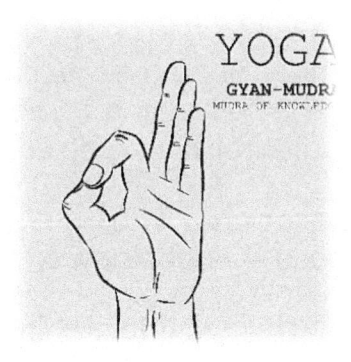

PRANA MUDRA

How to do it: the ring finger and little finger touch the thumb, while the middle and index fingers remain taut. It is mainly used to channel energy to the first chakra.

Meaning: This mudra is also known as the position of life, since it is able to direct vital energy throughout the body.

Benefits: this mudra is able to infuse us with energy during and after meditation. It also strengthens eyesight and the immune system.

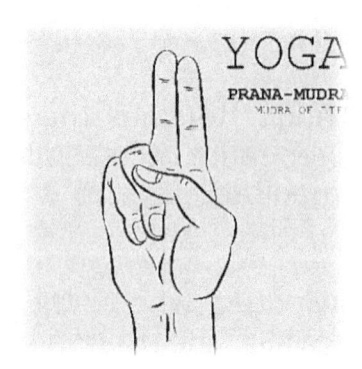

Vayu Mudra

How to do it: the index finger should be placed under the thumb, so that the latter exerts pressure. The remaining three fingers should be kept taut, but not too much (they should not cause discomfort).

Meaning: this mudra is associated with air and everything related to it: Ayurvedic medicine often uses this position to treat bodily dysfunctions.

What benefits it brings: this position is of great help for all physical problems related to a stagnation of air, for example, flatulence or abdominal bloating. Some Parkinson's patients have also found it beneficial in calming the symptoms of their condition.

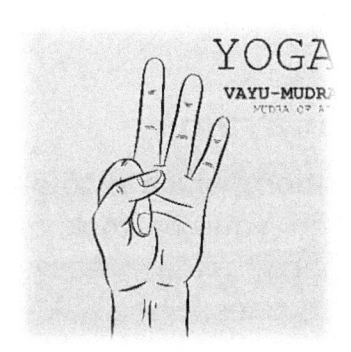

Apaan Mudra

How to do it: the middle and ring fingers touch the thumb, while the index and little finger remain slightly taut.

Meaning: This mudra correspond to purification, in the physical sense (being connected to digestion) and in the spiritual sense.

Benefits: this position is very useful in eliminating toxins from the body, especially indicated for digestion problems and beneficial for the heart and blood circulation.

The advice is to start with 10-15 minutes. The goal is to do 45 minutes of meditation, in progression, with the passage of time

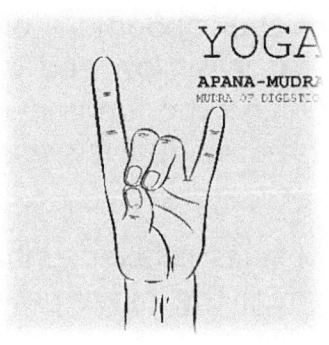

Ideal Position for Pranayama

You can sit in the lotus position, which is to place yourself on the floor, put something like a cushion on your buttock and bring your heels towards your butt, crossing your legs; all are easy. If you still don't have the flexibility to use the previous ones, Shoemaker Pose is the one you need.

You can also use a cushion to sit on. As a result, the hips are higher, the knees are lower, and the stability is greater. Another option, which is the one I recommend for the book at hand, is to use a chair to keep your back straight, which can prevent your legs from falling asleep if you spend a long time doing pranayama.

Types of Pranayama

In the sense of the type of breathing, Pranayama is divided into three types. I have named them before in this chapter and will now expand on them. Try these types of breathing and feel them inside you:

Abdominal Breathing

Abdominal breathing is the most common and is something we do unconsciously.

When you inhale, the lower lungs fill with air, which moves the diaphragm down, and you can see the abdomen expand. Pranayama involves controlling the breath so that it is slow and quiet. It should also be quiet, as this means that the air filling the lungs is drawn in slowly. If you catch yourself and/or hear your breathing, it is because it is too fast. Try to slow it down.

Keeping your abdominal muscles relaxed, inhale and exhale through your nose at all times. You can feel the movement by placing a hand on your stomach.

Thoracic Breathing

As you inhale like this, you will notice your ribs moving as your rib cage expands. To feel this breath as much as possible, contract your belly and inhale. Belly distension can be prevented by tensing the abdomen so that the part that expands is the thorax.

Clavicular Breathing

This is produced by filling the upper part of the lungs with air. You may not have heard of this breathing method, but if you watch closely, you will notice the very subtle movements of the clavicle.

When you inhale, raise your collarbone, but don't make any movement with your shoulders. Did you get that? I told you it is subtle, but it is also inefficient. It is mentioned only because it is important if the other two breathing movements accompany it.

When we do these three breathing types simultaneously, we do a complete breath, which is the pranayama instruction. Each type can fill the lung area with air, and if they are performed at the same time, we can make the lungs work to their maximum capacity.

The correct method of adjusting the breath is: first do abdominal breathing, then do chest breathing, and finally do clavicle breathing. When emptying the lungs, the order is reversed.

Dirga, Three-Part Breath

The purpose of Dirga is to make the abdomen expand like a balloon; it expands outward on the inhalation and retracts into the spine on the exhalation.

First, to practice Dirga, get into a comfortable position, either sitting in a chair or on a yoga mat. Sit up straight. Begin the exercise with a few normal breaths and observe as you inhale and exhale.

Next, inhale, focus on breathing slowly, and let your belly inflate like a balloon. Breathe in more air, filling and expanding the chest cavity. Finally, allow the air to come up through your chest and collarbone.

Now begin to exhale slowly. Release the air from the chest and collarbone first. Then slowly release the air from the chest cavity and abdomen. The abdomen should retract and move toward the spine until the exhalation is complete. Repeat the operation three times.

Bhastrika

This is another group of breathing techniques that make up the fourth branch of yoga, "Pranayama." This method is also based on breathing and is called fire breathing. The Bhastrika technique is similar to the previous one but with faster breathing. Also, in a rhythmic and sustained way, hold your breath for a few seconds before exhaling.

It is all a matter of practice until you get the exact accompaniment to practice with enough precision. This technique is previous to the technique called Kapalabhati, which is why they must be performed orderly because they are somehow related to each other.

Breathing is quite strong, similar to observing that of a person who has just run for a long time, i.e., short, deep breaths.

Nadi Sodhana

We are dealing with a cleansing breathing movement, which can cleanse the lungs directly through the breathing channels. This word comes from Sanskrit, where Nadi translates as "channel" and Sodhana translates as "purification."

Nadi Sodhana is a breathing technique practiced to purify the entire respiratory tract, especially the lungs.

Of all the breathing techniques or rules that make up the fourth branch of yoga, "Pranayama," it can be said that this is the most important, as it provides sanitation of the respiratory tract. In other words, after practicing this technique, the respiratory system will carry out the rest of the exercises without problems.

It is deep breathing, alternating and purifying in itself. But it should be clarified that all these breathing techniques can be harmful in some cases, for example, if people have certain types of disease, such as angina, asthma, or other ailments related to the respiratory tract or coronary arteries.

The technique consists of inhaling through the left nostril, exhaling through the right nostril, inhaling again through the right nostril and exhaling through the left nostril. Thus, one of the nostrils is covered alternately with the help of the thumb and ring fingers of the right hand.

Simhasana, Lion's Breath

Simhasana (Lion's Breath) is a powerful breath that can help you release depression. It is a different pose whose focus is on the breath.

You get into a comfortable position with good posture in a chair. First, inhale through your nose. Exhale, open your mouth wide, and say the word "ha."

Inhale again. On the next exhalation, in addition to saying "ha," stick out your tongue and point the tip of your tongue toward your chin.

Inhale again. Finally, exhale again with force, sticking out your tongue as you say "ha" and look at the ceiling. Do these three movements while exhaling and do three more breathing cycles.

Ujjayi

This Pranayama exercise should be done in this way:

- While sitting in the chair, perform the pranayama mudra and expel all the air from your lungs.
- The glottis (upper throat) is partially closed during inhalation. To do this, lower your head so that your chin is close to your chest. This inhalation should be slow.
- Now you should hold your breath.
- As we pointed out when talking about Pranayama Mudra, you should plug the right nostril and expel the air through the left nostril.

Kapalabhati

We are again facing another technique used in the fourth branch of Yoga, "Pranayama," the Kapalabhati. The first thing to do is to adopt the correct posture for this exercise. This should be the most common posture for yogis, sitting upright on the floor with legs crossed in the Buddha posture.

This practice is considered a warm-up before starting a more profound yoga practice. With this exercise, a deep cleansing of the brain is planned, through deep breathing and its known oxygenation, the brain cells are activated, and the mind becomes unequal.

The nostrils play an essential role in this exercise. It is through them that air must enter the lungs. The air that carries all the toxins must then be exhaled through the mouth.

This technique is ideal to slow down the flu process or to improve the patient's condition if the disease is already established.

- Begin by inhaling and exhaling the entire air until you are empty.
- Inhale to half your capacity.
- Exhale, exhale, exhale... Exhale rhythmically through the nose for 10-15 seconds, contracting the abdomen and contracting the navel on each exhalation.
- Inhale. Activate the bandhas and hold your breath as long as possible.
- Relax.
- Exhale.

Solar Breathing

Using the pranayama mudra, inhale the air through the right nostril and expel it through the left nostril, alternatively curving each nostril. Remember 5-10-10 cycles of breathing, but put a few seconds in the end, during which time you will still be without air, i.e., it will be 5-10-10-10-2.

Lunar Breathing

This technique is complementary to the previous Pranayama practice, in which you inhale through the left nostril and exhale through the right nostril.

Anulom Vilom

This exercise is done like this:

- Inhale through the left nostril, hold your breath, and exhale through the right nostril.
- Inhale through the right side, hold your breath, and breathe out through the left nostril.

With the above, you will have completed one cycle. Start again always inhaling on one side, holding the air, and exhaling on the other side. Then, this will be the side you inhale from the next time.

The fourth branch of yoga, "Pranayama" (regulation of breathing), is very important since through breathing, you can regulate the blood flow by activating the circulation, which in itself leads to greater oxygenation of the brain, thus allowing the brain to respond adequately to any stimulus.

As we all know, yoga is an ancient Indian teaching subject, which is composed of 8 branches. Each of these has its function and its rules or principles.

Pranayama is considered the fourth branch of yoga, which is based on breath control. The origin of the name is divided into two, "Prana," which means vital energy, and "Ayama," which means extension. The word originates from Sanskrit and harmonizes energy through breathing.

However, this branch consists of different techniques, and we can say that basically, these are known techniques: Ujjayi, Bhastrika, Kapalabhati, and Nadi Sodhana, among others we have just described. It is worth noting that each of these techniques has its benefits, and they all form a whole around the breath.

But now let's see what benefits the fourth branch of yoga, "Pranayama," brings to its practitioners.

- It activates circulation, allowing better cerebral perfusion.
- It can help people to improve their concentration.
- It brings great peace and tranquility to those who manage to focus on this crucial branch of yoga.
- It helps to cleanse the lungs by increasing the oxygen they stop receiving.
- It is crucial for the elimination of toxins through exhalation.
- It calms feverish states and restless minds through relaxation.
- It helps to cure certain ailments, especially those related to the mind and body.
- It helps discard negative thoughts and drives away bad emotions such as revenge, resentment, sadness, frustration, grief, or anger.
- It actively promotes cell regeneration.

- It brings an undeniable sense of well-being that can be felt almost immediately upon beginning a breathing exercise.
- It increases the amount of oxygen in the blood, with secondary benefits.

Knowing this, let's start doing the first chair yoga exercises, but first, we must warm up.

Savasana Pose

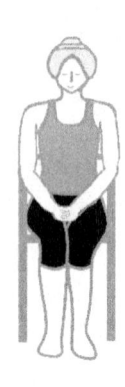

Chapter 2: Warm-up

Stretching has many advantages and can be done at any time with your doctor's approval.

Gently stretch your body to increase circulation and relieve muscle tension. Take advantage of the benefits of stretching and sustain the range of motion throughout the process. Before practicing chair yoga, it is very necessary to warm up so that every joint and muscle is ready for the process we will subject it to.

Benefits of Warming Up Before Chair Yoga

Studies have shown that stretching provides several benefits for wheelchair users and older adults around the world. Benefits include flexibility, improved circulation, stress relief, better posture and coordination, increased energy levels and joint range of motion, and reduced muscle tension.

Among the most common exercise concerns you may have are:

- What exercises and activities should you not do?
- How much exercise can you do per day and week?
- What types of exercises are recommended?
- What type of medication you take can influence your exercise routine?

Every person who does chair yoga may have illnesses and medical conditions that prevent them from doing more intense exercises. Discuss the best exercises for you with your doctor or physical therapist and find the best stretching options.

Warm-Ups You Can Do in a Chair

- The first time you do this, you should hold your left elbow with your right hand. Gently move your elbows behind your head until you feel a slight stretch in your shoulders or the back of your arms. Then repeat the same steps for the other arm.

- Hold your left elbow with your right hand and gently pull your elbow behind your head until you feel a full stretch. Then, gently lean to the side of your hips; stretch along the side of your upper body. Now repeat the same steps with the other arm.

- For this other step, raise your arms above your head with your palms facing up. Push your arm back a little and then up. Feel the stretch in your arms, back, and shoulders.

- For this exercise, keep your hips straight in a chair and turn your upper body to the right and left. Turn around so you can look over your shoulder. This exercise helps you stretch your sides and back.

- Fingers interlocked, palms out, arms extended in front of you at shoulder height. Extend your arms forward to stretch your shoulders, arms, upper middle back, wrists, fingers, and hands.

- This exercise requires gently bringing the elbows over the chest toward the opposite shoulder until a comfortable stretch is achieved.

- Gently bend forward to stretch the area from the neck to the lower back. Find a comfortable position and hold it for a minute or two. Then you sit down, put your hands on top of your thighs and push your upper body into an upright position.

- In the next exercise, you will pull your upper shoulders toward your earlobes and hold them for 5 to 8 seconds. Then relax completely and allow the shoulders to drop naturally. Perform the same movement repeatedly to relieve tension and stiffness in the shoulders and neck.

- Begin this next exercise with good posture in a chair. Tilt your head to the left as you drop your right shoulder. Repeat on the other side. With this exercise, you will stretch your neck.

- For this exercise, you will cross your fingers behind your head and keep your elbows out to the sides. Hold your upper body upright in the middle. Bring your shoulder blades together, creating tension through your upper back and shoulder blades. Hold the tension for 10–15 seconds, and then relax. Repeat this exercise several times.

- This exercise requires you to sit centered and upright while placing your fingers behind your head. Gently and carefully bring your head down until you feel a little stretch in the back of your neck. If you have a cervical spine injury, talk to your doctor before doing this.

- Bring one of your knees toward your chest until you feel a little stretch. Hold this position until the tension disappears. Then, extend the leg slowly until you feel a smooth, comfortable pressure. Repeat the exercise with the other leg.

For an older person or one with limited physical fitness to do physical exercise, these yoga techniques are necessary. They are designed to prepare the body to avoid injuries and other problems that physical activity can cause.

Remember that the warm-up should be done calmly, without forcing the muscles and joints. One of the main consequences of an inadequate warm-up is sprains, strains, and even joint lacerations.

Beyond that, a physical activity routine like this is excellent for improving coordination and improving your physical and mental health.

Neck Movements

You start by straight back. Relax all your muscles and let your back and legs be fully extended and loose. Once you adopt this posture, you have to move your head up and down with a calm rhythm, not with haste or abruptness.

This warm-up is usually done in 10 repetitions, and when you finish, you can repeat the exercise but moving your head from right to left.

After these 2 exercises, do the same but move your jaw from right to left, with your eyes looking straight ahead. Repeat the same number of times.

Older people must always look forward to avoiding possible dizziness, so we recommend that the person who performs them is supervised. Neck exercises provide flexibility to our muscles and help us to exercise the vestibular part, the part that helps us to regulate our balance and spatial control.

Tips for When You Exercise
- You may find it helpful to use a timer or watch to check that you have stretched enough.
- Breathe normally. Do not hold your breath while warming up or exercising.
- Exercise slowly and smoothly. Do not make quick or jerky movements.
- Look in a mirror as you move to ensure you are in the correct posture.
- Stop any exercise that causes pain, nausea, dizziness, swelling, or discomfort. If this happens, call your healthcare provider and inform him or her.

Practice 2 times a day for 3 months, and always warm up before you start. You may be able to move your shoulder and regain full neck movement in 3 months. If this happens, tell your healthcare provider if you can stop exercising. Also, keep your healthcare provider informed if you still cannot move your neck or shoulders after 3 months of doing these exercises.

Stretch Your Neck Diagonally and Upward

This is something you can do twice a day.
- Gently turn your head to look up and to the right.
- Place your right hand on your left cheek and chin. Apply a slight pre-squeeze so you can stretch a little more.
- Repeat this movement in the other direction.
- Hold each stretch for 30 seconds and then relax. Take 1 deep breath between each short repetition. Repeat the exercise 5 times on each side.

Diagonal Neck Stretch: Downward

You can do it 2 times a day.
- Gently turn your head to face downward and to the left.

- Put your left hand on your head. Then apply a little pressure to stretch a little more.
- Repeat this movement in the other direction.
- Hold each stretch for 30 seconds and then relax. Take 1 deep breath between each repetition. Repeat the exercise 5 times on each side.

Stretching the Neck Side

You can do it 2 times a day.

- Sit or stand with your right arm down.
- Put your left hand on top of your head.
- Gently tilt your head over your left shoulder to stretch the muscles on the right side of your neck.
- Repeat this movement in the other direction.
- Hold each stretch for 30 seconds and then relax. Take 1 deep breath between each repetition. Repeat 5 times on each side.

Pectoral Stretch in a Doorway

You can do this 2 times a day.

- Stand in the space of the open door.
- Put your hands and forearms shoulder-width apart on both sides of the door.
- Step forward gently until you feel a slight stretch in the front of your chest and shoulders. Keep your back straight, and your neck and shoulders relaxed.
- Hold the position for 30 seconds and then relax.
- With your arms at your sides, return to the starting position.
- Take 1 deep breath between each repetition. Repeat 5 times.

Chin Tuck

- Sit or stand with your back and head against the wall.

- Tighten your jaw and try to rest your neck against the wall. You will hold this position for 5 seconds and then relax.
- Return to the starting position.
- Take 1 deep breath between each repetition. Repeat the action 10 times.

Jaw Lowering

You can do it 2 times a day.

- Sit or stand in front of a mirror to see your face.
- Put the tip of your tongue behind your upper teeth.
- Slowly lower your lower jaw so that you open your mouth while keeping your tongue touching your upper jaw. Use a mirror to ensure you open your mouth evenly and do not move your jaw from side to side. Hold this position for 10 seconds, and then relax.
- Close your mouth.
- Take 1 deep breath after each repetition. Repeat 10 times.

Shoulder Exercise

For this part of the body, start by bringing the shoulders to the ears, and once they are as high as possible, slowly lower them. Repeat the movement 10 times in total. After the first exercise, we will bring the shoulders forward and backward, keeping the back and legs completely straight. Make circular movements to complete the shoulder warm-up routine, 10 forward and 10 backward.

These exercises will help you warm up your back and chest muscles, which are very important at this stage of life.

Exercises for Arms and Elbows

You must prepare the joints in this area for this physical exercise. In addition, without changing the straight-back posture, you will also do some exercises for arms and elbows.

Extend your arms at the elbows, then begin to raise them above the shoulders for a total of 10 repetitions. When you complete this exercise, do the same movement, but in a lateral way, that is, with the arms and elbows facing the sides of the body.

After these two exercises, take the position you had in the first exercise (arms bent at the elbows) and bring your arms down so that your elbows are close to your hips. This exercise allows you to open your hands and then close them, which is very positive for the coordination of the warm-up.

Exercises for the Back and Abdominal Area

Put your hands on your waist and start leaning your body forward and backward at the same pace, no matter how you lean. Do this ten times in total.

After this exercise, return to the starting position and try to put your hands as low as possible on your legs; you have to work your back as much as possible. Do this a total of 10 times in both directions, right and left.

Then raise your elbows and bring your palms together at the level of your head. In this position, then move your torso from side to side and fully straighten your legs.

It is important to do these movements by warming up this body area and tightening the abdomen.

Many of the most common exercises are trunk flexions, but these exercises can negatively affect the spine. Every time the trunk is flexed, it puts a lot of pressure on the lumbar spine, causing wear and tear of the discs and cervical pain due to improper performance of the movements.

For this reason, one must try to exercise, without affecting the spine and maintaining stability, with the help of a mat:

- With your back against the floor, legs bent, and feet flat on the floor, lift one knee and apply pressure with the opposite hand; leave the elbow extended while exhaling for about 4 to 5 seconds. Inhale as you lower your legs.

- Same as the previous exercise, but now you are going to lift both legs simultaneously, exhale and press with both hands for about 4 seconds.
- One way to work the lower back is to do those abdominal exercises called anti-extension, anti-flexion, and anti-rotation.

Exercises for the Legs

For a successful leg warm-up, you can perform a simulated run, that is, do the usual running movements. But these movements should be slow and not exaggerated. It is important to raise your arms and knees as high as possible.

The second exercise will consist of doing mini squats, which can be done more or less depending on the psychomotor skills of each person.

After the squat, return to the starting position (back and legs straight), bring the legs together, and keep them as far as possible from the body's center. It is essential to have a stationary leg on each incline so that both the left and right sides of the body are worked. You do this exercise a total of 10 times in both directions.

The last exercise focused on warming up the legs and working the biceps, quads, and hamstrings, which are essential parts of our body, especially as we age.

Bring one leg at a time, to hip height and, at the same time raise the heel. A total of 10 repetitions will do a good job of activating the lower half of your body.

With the heels up, let's do another running movement, this time without lifting the feet out of sleep and without exaggerating the leg movement.

Ankle and Foot Exercises

We will work the ankles to finish exercising the legs to avoid breaks or sprains. Lift the ankles and make circular movements inwards and outwards. Repeat this exercise 10 times in both directions. When working in the other direction, keeping one foot firmly on the ground is important.

These exercises will help prevent physical injuries that can occur during sports or certain activities. However, there are many aspects to consider, including the physical condition of the person doing the warm-up.

Warm-up Exercises for Arms and Back

The first activity you will do in this part of the warm-up is to bring your hands as far above your head as possible. Once you are at that point, try to hold for ten seconds. Warm up your muscles by repeating this exercise with both arms.

Then bring your arms forward and leave them at chin level, and once they are hard, try to hold for ten seconds.

Trunk Warm-up Exercises

After warming up your arms and back, it's time to start working the core, which is a fundamental part of our mobility during exercise.

In the first exercise, you will warm up using a chair. Grab the right armrest with both hands and lean your body to the right keeping your arms tense. Once in this position, try to stay on your side for about 10 seconds.

You should also use a chair to warm up your glutes and lower back. Hold the right side of the armrest with both hands to strain your lower back, and once you feel the tension in that area, try holding both sides for 10 seconds.

For the last warm-up exercise for the trunk, it is recommended to tie the hips to the chair to avoid falling. Once this safety "measure" is in place, try to keep your arms under your legs as much as possible. When you feel some tension, try to hold it for 15 seconds.

Injuries That Can Occur Due to a Bad Warm-up

I will never get tired of repeating that the warm-up is very important. Even though these are chair yoga exercises, you need to take care of every movement in the process. Let's see what could happen to you.

Sprain

In some stages of life, major sprains often occur during physical activity. This setback is often very detrimental when you have some health conditions, as it becomes more difficult for the body to heal tears in your ligaments as time goes on.

Muscle Cramps

Muscle cramps occur when our muscles contract from fatigue, causing intense pain that usually lasts for a few minutes.

Fibrillar Rupture

A poor warm-up can lead to fibrous and torn muscles. These injuries are caused by the tearing of muscle fibers due to overstretching. These tears are very common in a sedentary lifestyle and strain the muscles to the point of breaking fibers. After such a tear, the person should rest for 2 to 3 weeks before exercising again.

Tendonitis

Tendonitis is technically the inflammation of a tendon, usually caused by repetitive movements.

This is a common problem in older people as their muscle tissue ages, sometimes manifesting as tendinitis in elbows, shoulders, hands, etc. Arthritis can also be caused by taking excessive medications often used to alleviate some degenerative diseases.

Adults need to be physically active, especially when they reach a certain age, or when they have been incapacitated by an operation or medical condition, to avoid diseases such as osteoarthritis or tendonitis.. A World Health Organization (WHO) report shows the importance of physical activity on older adults' cardiorespiratory and muscular systems. In this sense, exercise can also help prevent diabetes and high blood pressure and improve bone mass. In addition, encouraging people to be physically active helps their spatial control and combat loneliness.

The report published by the World Health Organization explains that moderate exercise for an average of 1:30 hours per week or vigorous exercise for about 75 minutes per week is the most appropriate. It is very necessary to perform different activities to achieve active aging.

Chapter 3: Beginners Program

Let's do some of the simplest and most practical poses to start working on your body from scratch.

- Since the sets in this sequence will be done with the support of a chair in a seated position, you should make sure that the chair you are looking for is comfortable, with a flat base, and not so thick with padding. You should also choose a chair with a low height so that you can touch the floor effortlessly to promote proper blood flow.

- Start by sitting down, placing your legs on either side of the legs of the chair, and stretching your spine upward until you are comfortable. Never go beyond your comfort zone.

- Bring your palms to the namaste position, to your chest near your heart chakra, and close your eyes.

- Start feeling the freshness of the breath flowing through your nostrils as you seek to fill your belly and lungs.

- You may have to take several breaths to understand this; make sure your breathing is also slow and steady.

- As time goes on and you fulfill your responsibilities, it is time to focus from deep within and start this slow connection. As you breathe, take a moment to understand and answer questions that fill you with worry, such as who, why, and what.

- Sit and take about 6 or more breaths and put a smile on your face; let the muscles be relaxed and calm.

Neck Wheels

- After a good start with the deep breathing round and calming the nerves in the entry exercise, open your eyes, rub the palms of your hands together to generate warmth, and hold them over your eyes for a while.

- Then inhale and bring your neck up and back as far as you feel comfortable, then exhale fully. Then inhale, bring your neck to your chin, and exhale all the way out.

- Do this neck exercise in 2 rounds while breathing 2 times per round.

- Make sure that you do not force the body and the movement by trying to coordinate the breathing with the movement. If the breath and movement do not synchronize, ensure you still breathe well.

- Depending on how comfortable you are, you can choose to close your eyes.

- Sit in the chair so that you feel comfortable, keeping your neck relaxed.

The Same Exercise as Above Is Viewed from a Different Angle
- Now direct the neck from the center to the right shoulder as you release the air and return to the center.

- As you inhale and exhale, bring the neck from the center to the left shoulder and return to the center.

- Repeat this neck movement from the center to the shoulders and back; if everything is going well, close your eyes and relax your body while continuing the movement.

- Reducing and opening blockages around the top helps the prana to flow smoothly to the brain, so you will have a calm and relaxed mind.

- While these movements look simple, they do wonders for the nervous system when you are done with the breathing process.

Exercise Variation to Relieve Aches and Pains
- Now, stand in the center and relax for a few breaths. If your head feels uncomfortable from the neck movement, breathe deeply through both nostrils.

- Now, slowly, while breathing, move your neck to the right and the left for two rounds, breathing twice in each round.

- Be sure not to strain the body and movement by trying to coordinate the breathing with the movement. If the breath and exercise are not synchronized, ensure you are breathing correctly.

- The idea of rotating here is to release any tension that has built up around both the neck and shoulders, doing as they say, "take the weight off the shoulders." Tension and stiffness in the neck and shoulder blades can cause headaches and sleep deprivation.

- If you follow the movement and close your eyes, you will connect with the world around you.

Shoulder Circles

- Place your neck facing forward.

- Now place your palms on your shoulders near the base of your neck, bend your elbows, fully extend your spine and sit up straight.

- Turn your arms in a circle, forward and backward, while bending to the right and to the left twice, breathing twice each time you make a circle.

- If you find it difficult to raise your arms that high, just bend your hands at the elbows and use your shoulders to rotate

- This stretch aims to keep your shoulders, elbows, and wrists active and reduce any symptoms associated with arthritis or osteoporosis.

Lateral Stretch From Chair

- Start with shoulder and arm rotations, relax your hands, close your eyes, and slowly breathe in and out.

- Then inhale and lift your right arm as far as you can to the left as you slowly tilt your chest and neck to the left.

- Exhale completely, then inhale again and repeat for a few seconds without stopping breathing.

- Now inhale and extend your right arm and lower it towards the chair, then exhale so that you relax your neck and shoulders.

- You will repeat this arm movement, in a lateral stretch posture sitting on the chair.
- Make sure you are well balanced and don't do it too far to the left, lest you lose your balance.

Lateral Stretch Exercise Holding Onto the Chair

- Release your left arm and repeat while keeping your right arm down to hold the chair.
- This stretch aims to gently open your heart muscle, which helps you breathe better.
- Move slowly and keep your balance.

Twists in a Chair

- Rest from the side stretching postures and now relax in a comfortable seat.
- Then, while holding onto the chair with both hands, inhale and slowly twist to the right, moving your torso from the hips to the rest of your body, facing backward, and exhaling fully.
- Now, you will turn while sitting to the left, holding your breath for a moment, then relax, inhale slowly, and return to the starting position and repeat.
- Do 2 rounds to the right, 2 or more breaths per round.

Activating the Torso

- Release, and once you are in the center, turn to the left by twisting your torso.
- Keep your balance as you turn, make sure your body doesn't move, and breathe gently.
- Torso twists serve to activate the spine, thus increasing the flow of prana from below. These twists also help to maintain flexibility in the hips and shoulders.

Expanding the Chest

- After doing the torso twists, return to the center and relax your spine and shoulders, keeping your breathing calm and slow.

- Now you are going to inhale, sitting on the chair with your hands behind you, and lift your chest up and out while you go up your neck a little bit and try to look up.

- You should do this for two or three rounds. Connect your body movements and enjoy the stretch in your chest and lower spine.

- This is an excellent way to activate the body's glands while keeping your balance in check. It helps you breathe more deeply and also helps the digestive system function, and deep breathing keeps the mind calm and focused.

Hands Up

- Relax and sit comfortably after the chest expansion and take several breaths.

- Now, inhale and raise your arms above your head, open your chest, and fully extend your shoulders and arms.

- Exhale once while remaining seated and breathe with your hands up for 1 or 2 breaths or as long as possible.

- If you find it challenging to raise your arms, you can raise one arm at a time or raise both arms as high as you can, even with your elbows bent.

- Raise your arms above the level of your heart to help your heart pump better, which is great for stress management and a healthy heart.

- If you can, close your eyes and focus on yourself. Enjoy the peace, and concentrate on the sounds coming from within, as your arms will partially block your ears.

Head Up

- Inhale and extend your arms upward. Move forward while flexing your hips, then lower your arms toward your legs and exhale the air fully.

- This pose, rising from the chair, is similar to Uttanasana, where the hips bend to move forward. Here, you should look upward by bending the neck while the hands comfortably reach for the legs or feet.

- Here, leaning on the back of the chair and with your head raised, you will compress the abdomen, which will help you with the functioning of the internal organs.

Internal Organ Function

This position helps you have better digestion, fewer urinary tract infections, and better insulin balance.

- Make sure there is no pressure on your chest or abdomen as you move forward, and if you feel comfortable, hold this position by taking 4 slow, deep breaths.

- Inhale and lift your torso so that you are balanced and relaxed. You can do this posture often, with your arms raised on the back of the chair, hands up, exhale into the chair, and head up.

Pigeon Pose

- After practicing the previous exercise, relax and sit comfortably.

- Now inhale and lift your right leg a little with your hands and place it on your left thigh where it will sit comfortably.

- The flexion of the hips and knees will benefit from this position, as it helps to keep them healthy and flexible.

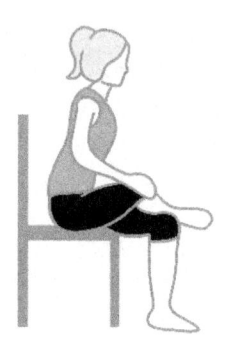

- Once you are comfortable, sit up as straight as possible and take 2 breaths. If you find it complex to bring your leg up and over the other leg, lift your right leg and try to hug it for a few seconds, then slowly release it.

Lunge Variation

- Lift the right leg off the chair and press the right thigh toward the chest.

- If you have difficulty bending your thighs toward your chest due to the heaviness of your body and abdomen, use your hands to support your thighs or use a yoga strap comfortably.

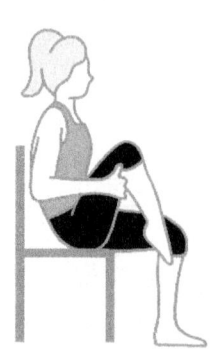

- Moving your knees by flexing your hips keeps your joints active and healthy and helps you recover quickly after a fall if you are injured.

- Hold the chair pose with the low lunge variation for about 2–3 breaths; you can repeat the pose after you release.

Sitting With Hands on Chest

- Now that you come out of the lunge variation pose sit up to relax your arms, shoulders, chest, and lower back.

- Place your hands on your chest, close your eyes, and breathe calmly to connect.

- Hold the position for approximately 6 breaths or as needed by the body.

Cactus Arms

- Once you are relaxed, raise your arms to shoulder height and extend them out to the sides as you bend your elbows and feel the stretch in your chest.

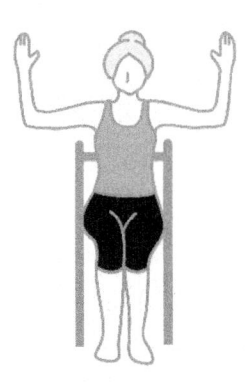

- Inhale and open your arms to expand your chest while looking straight ahead, keeping your spine extended or straight.

- Sitting in an armchair with your arms in a cactus-like position, extend your arms outward, helping to draw more air into your lungs so they are fresh and active.

- Hold that position for 2–3 breaths, then inhale again, bring your arms back, and sit comfortably.

- Repeat if you feel good and comfortable.

Healing Plantar Fasciitis

As we age, our feet become weaker and weaker, and blood circulation decreases due to decreased physical activity.

Therefore, taking care of the soles of your feet is key as we age. To keep all the nerves of the foot active, massage the inside of the foot gently; using a soft ball helps to apply pressure to the acupuncture points of the foot.

- First, put a ball under your left foot, sit comfortably, and roll the ball around; make sure the ball gently massages the sole of your foot.
- This ball massage will help soothe the pain and swelling if someone suffers from plantar fasciitis.
- In addition, it is a good method for improving Qi (vital energy) and blood while activating essential acupuncture points on the soles of the feet.
- Get comfortable and keep rolling the ball for about 45 seconds or more.

Healing Foot Pain

Take the ball off the left foot, place it under the right foot, and gently massage it with the ball's movement.

Hamstring Stretch

- So that you can keep your feet strong and with good circulation, you will follow with a gentle leg massage.
- Get a yoga strap, or a towel, wrap it around your left foot, tighten it, and hold the other end in your hand.
- You can ask someone else to help you put the strap on your foot.
- Hold the other end of the strap, inhale, and lift your left foot off the floor and up, extending your leg.
- Pull the straps toward you, raise your legs while trying to keep them perpendicular to your hips, and lower your back into the chair.

- Lift your leg when you feel comfortable, hold for 2 or 3 breaths or more if possible, and stay calm.

Here Is Another Variable You Can Do
- Loosen and remove the strap, put it on the right foot, and do the same movement.
- Leg lifts with straps help you have support in your calves and hamstrings; it allows them to contract without putting pressure on your lower back and glutes.
- Chair hamstring stretches will also help you feel sciatica to some extent.
- Hold this stretch for 2 or 3 breaths; then allow the rest of your body to relax and calm down.

Cat and Cow
- Relax out of the hamstring stretch pose of the strapped chair, and now take a few breaths and make sure your hips are correctly positioned in the chair and that your body is centered and relaxed.

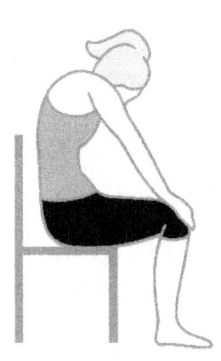

- Inhale, bring your chest up and your shoulders back to cow pose.

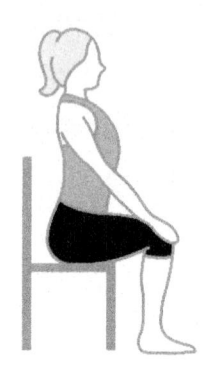

- Exhale and contract the chest, shoulders, and face, closing the jaw and looking to contract the abdominals.

- Repeat this movement for about 4 rounds, concentrating on the breath.

- This movement of the spine helps the body eliminate unwanted toxins and helps keep the internal organs healthy and in good condition.

- Release and relax by moving the body inward and resting your entire back on the chair. Sit up straight and close your eyes to calm your mind.

Hand Chest

These are some of the basic chair sequences created for people starting yoga; now just focus on breathing.

Sit comfortably in the middle, and align your face, shoulders, and chest. Now close your eyes and begin to feel the breath slowly pass through your nostrils.

After you do a few rounds here, start practicing Bhramari Pranayama. As you inhale, close your eyes with each finger, then exhale slowly, close your mouth, and make a sound.

The sound production is done at the back of the soft palate, where the mouth is closed to emit the sound like a bee. There, vibrations are created with each exhalation to calm the nervous system gradually.

Along with this breathing, the nerves that are in the neck, chest, head, and brain are calming down, thus relaxing the whole body.

You can do this exercise 8 to 10 times with each exhalation. Be aware of any kind of effort that may occur during exhalation, i.e., if you feel your heart rate increase with this exercise, and relax while breathing.

Close your eyes, rub the palms of your hands together to generate heat, and place them over your eyes for comfort. You can do the above sequence four times a week or more, as you can in your condition. Be sure to see a new you each time you do it. The new you should help you stay calm and detach from the outside world.

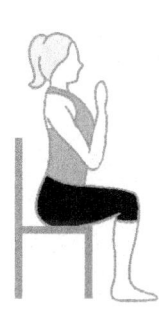

Chapter 4: Intermediate Program

When you've managed to do the basic poses, you're ready to move on to the others. Following a ritual as in the first one, we'll go from easy to intermediate in this chapter.

Mountain Chair Pose

- Begin the rectus muscle separation repair exercise by placing yourself in a chair with your feet on the floor, hands on your thighs, back straight, and eyes closed.

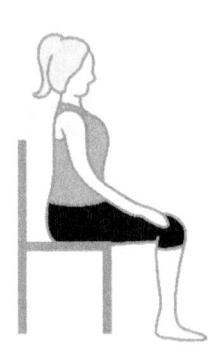

- Once seated, start breathing. Take about 2 breaths.

- Then, place your palms on your body (right hand on your belly, left hand on your chest) and notice your breathing. Much of the healing of the straight muscle stretches (and simple yoga postures) comes from awareness of the breath and connection to the body's movement.

- Focus on the movement of your belly and chest as you breathe. Hold that position for about 10 breaths.

Expanding Chest

Remember that your breathing should be slow and controlled throughout the exercise.

- Release your hands and place them behind you as you pull the lower end of the chair back.

- It is time to inhale, hold, and exhale. Then inhale and exhale again. Repeat this for about 6 breaths.

- When breathing, use your upper abdominal muscles, as this will help you repair the separation of the rectus muscle.

- Be sure not to pull your chest too much. Inhale and exhale slowly and consciously. The idea here is simply to use your upper abdominal muscles. Stay here for about 8 breaths.

- Make sure your feet are firmly on the floor and your thighs are firmly on the chair.

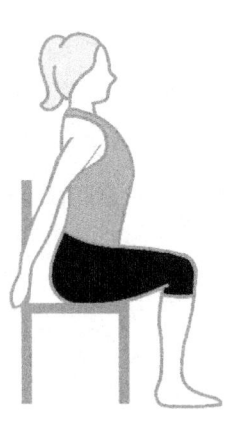

Torso Circles

- Now sit up straight and breathe.

- Next, place your hands on your lower abdomen, palms on either side of your belly.

- You will inhale and start doing torso circles on the chair, moving from right to left. Clasp your hands together and observe how your lateral abdominals work. Press your palms deep into your sides.

- Rotate clockwise and then counterclockwise in a slow circle. You will repeat the circle 3 times per side. Together that will be 6 circles (6 breaths).

- You will open and exhale as you exhale; focus on exhaling for a long time. Make a sound at that moment.

- Exhale through the open mouth so that you release the tension in the spine and, through this movement, make a conscious effort to breathe.

Floating on the Chair

- To continue the exercise above, sit down, raise your arms above your head, and release the air.

- Inhale again and assume the chair position, lifting the buttocks. Then exhale through your mouth and sit down.

- For a lighter exercise, rest your arms on the chair. Inhale and push your arms and buttocks up by contracting your abs. Then breathe and return to the starting position.

- Repeat 6 times (12 breaths); inhale while sitting, and exhale while standing. Bend your knees without over-tightening or extending your arms.

- Alternatively, place your hands on your belly and do the same movement.

Knees and Head Down

- Start with the seated low lunge variation chair exercise, relax, and rest.

- Follow the same instructions for the chair pose variation above, and practice with your head down.

- Bring your thighs up towards your face and rest your forehead on your knees.

- Keep inhaling and exhaling as you count to 6 (6 breaths).

- Don't overdo it when pressing and stretching. Exhale forcefully if necessary.

- Relax and repeat 6 times (6 breaths) with the other leg.

Camel Pose

- Sitting on a chair, resting your hands on the chair behind you, inhale and draw the shoulder back, then arch the torso with chin up, making the camel pose. Exhale and relax your body. Repeat 3 times (6 breaths).

- Place a folded towel or a blanket on the floor. Kneel down with the chair behind you. Place your arms back, hands on the chair and feet underneath it. Arch while repeating the camel pose movement applied while seated. Repeat 3 times with 6 breaths. Release and relax on the chair.

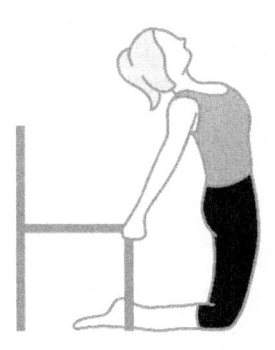

Table Pose and Knee-to-Nose Flow Pose

- Now, you stand in front of the chair.

- Lean forward and rest your hands on a chair. Inhale and bend your right leg placing your right knee between your hands. Release the air, and extend your leg backward.

- Repeat about 4 times (4 breaths) while moving slowly and exhaling through your mouth.

- When you extend your leg behind you, ensure it is not too straight.

- Relax and repeat with the other leg.

- If you feel confidence, in turn, place one hand on your belly as you move down to coordinate the movement of your abdominal muscles.

Tied Angle Pose

- Sit on the floor near a chair (relaxed posture) to perform this pose.

- Put your arms on the chair in front of you and slightly stretch your torso.

- Relax and focus on the movement of your spine as you breathe.

- Make sure that the distance between you and the chair does not stretch your abdomen too much.

- Relax by breathing fully, about 6 times.

- While yoga postures are used to treat separations of the rectus muscles, they can also help with conditions such as back pain, indigestion, and weak pelvic floor muscles.

Squat Against the Wall in a Standing Position

- Now approach the wall.

- Standing with your feet about 3 inches from the wall, place your palms on the wall behind you. Make sure your lower back is against the wall.

- Inhale and slowly lower yourself down while resting your back against the wall, then bend your knees into a squat.

- Stay like this for about 1 breath, then inhale again. Repeat 3 times.

- Inhale and lower. Exhale as you lower into a squat. Inhale and exhale in this position. Inhale and come up, exhale, and relax.

- This is a great way to work your abdominals while supporting your back. You can exhale with your mouth open, as this will ensure a full exhale.

Back-to-Back Chair Pose

- Now, you can move a little away from the wall.
- Ask someone for help (if you don't have it, practice on the wall). Do the chair pose back-to-back with the other person.
- You will keep your elbows locked while your backs face each other.
- Breathe out and down and stay in that position for about 6 breaths. You can repeat 3+3 times.

The Elevator

You can repeat this pose with a partner or do it alone.

- Perform the elevator pose while ex-pulling yourself up. You stand with the other person holding hands with your feet 1 foot apart.
- Release the air and lower down, bending your knees. Make sure your knees are comfortable and that the distance between the two of you is not too great so that your abdominal muscles are not stretched too much.
- Hold for about 6 breaths. This can also be divided into 3+3 if you want to relax in the middle of each set.
- In case you need the help of another person, they will be at your side to lift you gently or support you in case you do not have enough strength.

Constructive Rest

- Take some time away from practicing standing yoga postures and lie down on your mat or bed in a constructive resting position.
- Place your hands at your sides and breathe deeply for 2 rounds to relax.

- Continuing with this exercise, now place your right hand on your chest and the other on your belly.

- Observe the movement of the abdomen and chest and begin to breathe consciously for 8 rounds. Breathing should be slow, deep, and prolonged.

- When you inhale, ensure there is no additional pressure on your abdomen; be very careful.

Constructive Rest, Arms Crossed

- Now, cross your arms and bring them close to your chest as if hugging yourself.

- Feel your lower ribs and, as you breathe, push your ribs with your hands.

- Taking care of the upper part of the abdomen (closer to the ribs) is considered a way to start repairing the separation of the rectus muscle.

- Hold this position for about 6 deep, slow, deliberate breaths.

Supine Extension Pose

- Practice this pose while still lying on the mat on your back, with crossed legs, to continue with the constructive rest poses.

- Take a breath and raise your left arm above your head while stretching your right leg down, pushing your heel towards the floor.

- Hold this variation of the supine recline stretch for about 1 breath, then release the air to return the arms and legs to their original position.

- Take a breath, return to the posture, and hold for 1 breath. Repeat approximately 4 times (8 breaths), alternating arms and legs.

- Control your breathing as you move your arms and legs up and down. You can open your mouth to exhale completely.

Half Wind Release Pose

- Start from a constructive rest position, on the rug, take a breath, and bring the right leg up.

- Breathe, press the knee closer to you, bending it and support the right thigh with your hand. In the airflow, bring your thigh toward your chest as you inhale and exhale.

- Repeat this push and hold, then release and lower it to release the airflow 6 times (6 breaths), both legs.

- Get into a pose where you relax your abdominal muscles without stretching them too much. This also helps you control digestion, soothe back pain and keep your pelvic floor muscles active and strong.

- The exercise can also be performed on a chair as shown in the drawing (next page).

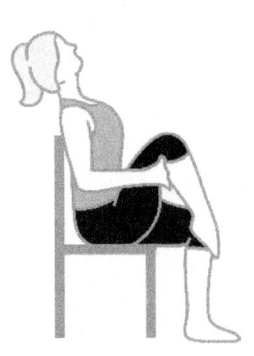

Happy Baby Pose

<u>On the mat</u>:

- Get into the constructive rest position.

- Breathe in and raise first your right leg and then your left leg while bending at the knee. Breathe in and stretch your arms out to grasp your big toes.

- Grasp the toes and slowly pull the thighs toward the chest without pushing too hard and make sure the abdominals are not overloaded with the contraction.

- In this pose, the full contraction of the abdominal muscles causes the correct relaxation of the rectus muscle.
- Hold for about 6 breaths. Tighten your stomach as you release the air without pressing your thighs against your chest.

<u>On the chair:</u>
- Sitting mid-chair, lean forward slowly by extending your arms down. With the fingers of your hands grasp your big toes, creating a slight contraction for 6 breaths.

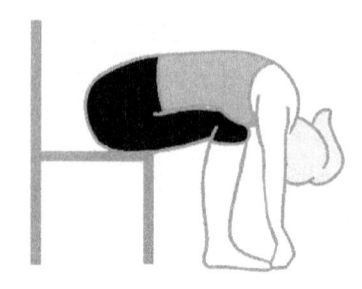

The Eagle Pose
- For the Eagle pose, sit away from the back of the chair. Take a breath.
- Cross the left leg on the right, that is connected to the floor.
- You find that the left foot stays out towards the outside edge of your right calf. Try to sneak it towards the inside.
- Lift your arms, lengthen up and reach up as high as you can.
- Let the arms open into goddess arms, draw the shoulders back and open through the heart space (Cactus pose).
- Bring the forearms together and cross them putting the left one on the right forearm.
- Hand palms will be open facing outwards. Hold three to five breaths.
- Repeat on the other side.

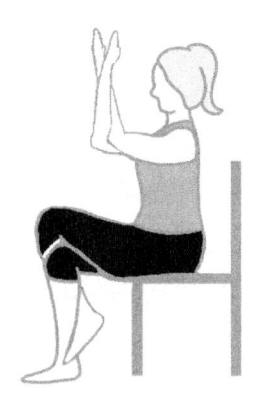

Reinforcing Happy Baby Pose
- In a constructive resting position, spread your feet apart and place a pillow on your stomach.
- Place one end of the pillow away from your body and place the other end on your chest.
- Inhale and lift your legs up and over the headrest, ankles wobbling.
- Hold Happy Baby Pose for about 6 breaths, relaxing the body. Make sure you feel relaxed when your spine touches the floor or bed. Watch the belly move and the head push but keep your breathing under control.

Squat to the Wall
- Standing with your back to the wall, less than a step away, rest your back and touch the floor with your toes.
- Slide down by bending your knees until you get into a "comfortable" sitting position. Then come back up.
- Do this 4 times. It is important to pace the breath in the ascent and descent phases.
- Alternatively, you can sit on a chair, facing the wall, slightly apart, resting your hands on the wall, above your head.
- Push with your legs and abdomens to stand up, levering with your hands.

- Return to a sitting position and relax. Repeat 4 times.

Side Bridge
- A challenging chair yoga pose is to practice the side bridge pose with your elbows bent.
- Get into a constructive resting position and turn to the left. Then place your right hand on the chair seat, in front of your chest and inhale.
- Exhale. Place your left elbow on the chair, moving with the left hip towards the edge of the chair, let your body weight partially rest on it.
- Stretch your legs while trying to lift your chest by pushing with your left forearm and right hand, placed on the seat.
- You can place your right hand on your side and a cushion on the chair.
- Stay like this, breathing very slowly and calmly. It is good to exhale through your mouth, as this ensures you do not hold your breath.
- Hold this position for 4 breaths as long as it is comfortable for you or for as long as possible. Then switch to the other side.
- This is a good position to keep your abdominal muscles contracted and not put too much pressure on them. Notice how your upper body gains strength, which is vital for keeping your abdominal muscles tight strong.

Garland Pose
- Stand with your feet hip-width apart, facing the chair.
- Hold your spine straight. Now sit comfortably with your hands resting on the chair, on a yoga block (you can put a blanket over it if you find it uncomfortable) and keep your spine straight. Take inspiration from the figures.

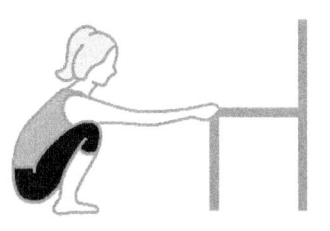

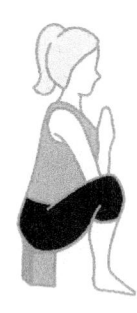

- Stay like this and notice how your belly moves, and your abdominal muscles as you breathe. Connecting with your body is the foundation (cannot be emphasized enough!) of every yoga posture practice.
- Stay in this position for 6–8 breaths.

Hugs, Twists, and Turns

- Relax and sit down.
- Cross your arms around your chest and hug yourself tightly. As you do so, feel your rib cage with the palms of your hands.
- Inhale and move your torso from right to left (without twisting), moving with your breath.
- Next, perform a relaxed hug, toward the hips and push the palms of the hands toward your belly.
- Just remember not to twist your body. Do this while executing 6 breaths.

Half Easy Pose and Half Forward Bend Pose

- Performing the half-forward bend pose to where you feel relaxed, release and stretch to allow a slight forward bend in the torso. Slightly bend your knees to descend; do this as far as possible.

- This posture helps to calm tight muscles in the lower back and contracted abdominal muscles.

- Hold for about 6 breaths and close your eyes. Connect and stay calm and relaxed. With this pose, you also work the pelvic floor muscles.

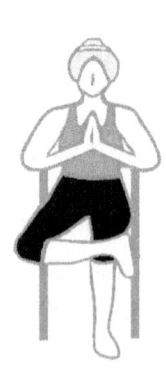

Broken Wings Pose

- Place your feet on the floor near the chair while bending your knees.

- Put your palms on either side of your belly. Get into broken wings pose.

- Contract your shoulders and chest as you inhale and push your hands as you exhale. Imagine physically bringing the sides of your abdominal muscles closer together.

- Stay like this for 6 breaths or more. You can also practice for 6 breaths, first relaxing and then repeating.

- This is a great way to connect your body while tightening your muscles.

Pose With Folding Blanket Blocks

Finish your yoga sequence with the relaxation method to follow here:

- Sit down and place a folded blanket block on your legs.

- Sit with your legs apart (not too far apart) bend over toward the folded blanket providing the necessary support for your chest, face, arms, stomach, and legs as far as you feel comfortable in this position.

- Breathe gently and hold this posture for about 3 minutes.

Alternatively, choose any relaxing yoga pose. I chose this variation specifically to calm the breath and relax all the back muscles.

Chapter 5: Advanced Program

If you already want to start an advanced program where you can work in different positions, in this chapter, you can start from the basics of warm-up and elementary postures to advanced and challenging ones.

Mountain Chair

- Sit on a chair with your feet forcefully on the ground.
- Place your hands on your knees, stretch your spine upwards, inhaling and detaching from the backrest.
- Close your eyes and exhale slowly, deeply, and then relax.
- Perform this exercise12 times, breathing slowly with a broad smile on your face.
- Stay positive, smile with each inhalation, and energize your body. Exhale completely to bring out the antioxidants that help boost your immune system.

- A cushion can support your back and keep your spine comfortable.

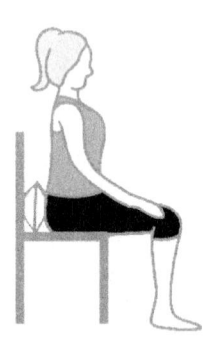

-

Neck Bends

- Start with the Tadasana pose, namely with the body straight, arms extended downwards, and palm forward then do the neck bending exercises.

- Inhale and slowly tilt your head back, stretching your neck.

- Release the air, tilt your head forward, and lock with your chin.

- Move up and down with the breathing process and breathe about 6 times.

- Take your time, and do not overdo it. In this exercise, concentrate on bringing the thoughts to your throat. This exercise can be done dynamically or by taking 2 breaths per pose.

- As you listen, immerse yourself in the comfort of your body. Remember also that communicating with your body is the best way to know if everything is working.

Tadasana Pose   Head Back 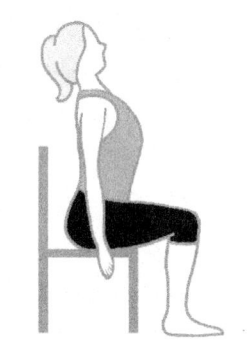   Head Forward

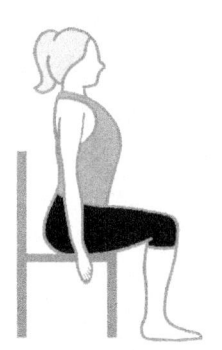

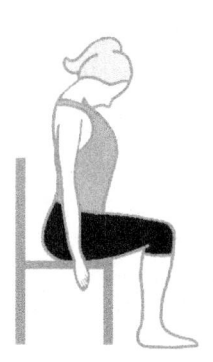

Turning the Neck

Now follow with a neck roll.

- Take a breath, turn your head to the right, and stretch the sides of your neck.

- Release the air and come back to the center. Take a breath and turn to the left.

- Breathe out and return to the center. Breathe in and repeat this movement for 6 rounds.

- Take slow, steady, deep breaths. The choice between a dynamic or static movement is yours, depending on the comfort of your neck and shoulders.

Cat Pose

- Relax and return to the mountain pose to calm yourself and connect with the breathing process.
- Take a breath, expand your chest, and slightly tilt your head and chin back.
- Release the air, bend your chest and shoulders inward, and touch your chin to your chest.
- Move dynamically in the chair between Cat and Cow poses. Smile and breathe positively as you do this.
- Practice this 6 times with the breathing process.

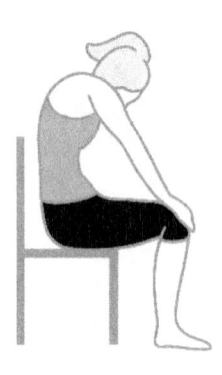

Cobra Pose

- Sit and relax in the center of the chair with your spine straight.
- Put your arms behind you so that you support yourself with the back of the chair and, as you inhale, lift your chest and shoulders to look up.
- Release the air and stay in the chair; feel the stretch in your neck and upper chest.

- Smile and repeat the movements for 6 breaths; take slow, deep breaths. Each time you exhale, feel your body stretch.
- Release, relax and repeat for a second round of 6 breaths.

This posture allows energy to flow slowly down the throat, which helps restore lost voice and energy.

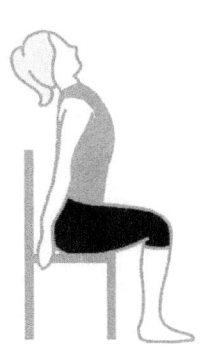

Chair Twist

- Stay in the chair, relaxed.
- Take a breath, put your right foot behind your left foot. Placing your left hand on right leg, put your right hand on the floor.
- Release the air and raise your head on the left.
- Get into the position and move your neck dynamically down as you exhale; then bring it up as you inhale. Hold the position by taking 6 breaths on the right side.
- Then, hold the position with the head and neck elevated for 6 breaths. Or you can do the movements with both sides alternately.
- You must choose what works best for you rather than overstretching and causing more pain and discomfort.
- Release and repeat the movement on the other side for 6 breaths.

Volcano Pose

- After performing several seated exercises for the neck and shoulders, now it's time to stand up.

- Start by inhaling and raising your arms above your head, touching fingers.

- Release the air and watch your fingers. Hold the volcano pose for about 6 breaths, otherwise move your arms up and down alternately, keeping a dynamic breath.

- With this pose, you fill your body with energy and antioxidants. This connection will be of great help in the healing process.

- Moving your arms or shoulders in any pose is not just about gaining strength and flexibility; it is about absorbing the earth's energy so that you are steady, confident, and happy.

Standing Rolling Down

- Follow with something challenging by doing the sequence from the standing pose to rolling down.

- From the mountain pose, take a breath and raise your upper back upward. Release the air, drop your shoulders, lock your chin with your chest, and look down.

- Take a breath, exhale, and slowly lean forward as your shoulders and neck rotate. To finish, exhale completely, pushing toward to the floor and lower your head.

- Do this forward fold for about 6 rounds, coordinating the breathing process.

- Take a breath, lift the body backward, lock the chin and rotate the shoulders. Release the air and return to mountain pose.

- This is a great exercise to stretch, contract, and activate the throat and neck. Don't forget to smile and feel the flow of energy.

Child's Table Pose

- Position yourself on a mat, kneel with your legs and toes touching.
- Rest your buttocks on your heels, exhaling.
- Bend the torso down, resting on the thighs with the arms extended forward, the forehead and palms on the floor.
- While inhaling, lift the torso forward, bringing the head in line with the hands, creating the shape of a table.
- You can hold the position while breathing 6 times or do this alternately, inhaling and exhaling.
- Before you work on doing it, dynamically or holding a longer posture, you should be clear about how comfortable you feel or how comfortable it is to breathe.

The expansion and contraction of the throat are stimulated along with the back of the spine and the chest area.

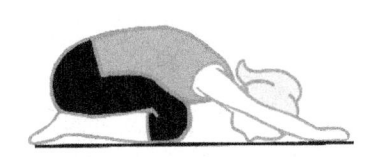

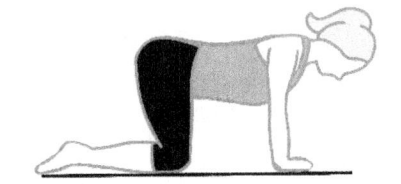

Needle Pose

- Release and relax into a table pose. Continue from there, leaving the Bolster in the middle of the body.

- Take a breath and slowly raise your left arm with your right arm extended forward.

- Release the air, bring the left arm, passing inward, to the right side and resting left shoulder and cheek on bolster.

- Rest and hold this position for 6 breaths.

- Take a breath and release slowly. Then repeat on the other side for 6 more breaths.
- You can do this with a dynamic flow, making sure your neck and shoulders are not tense.

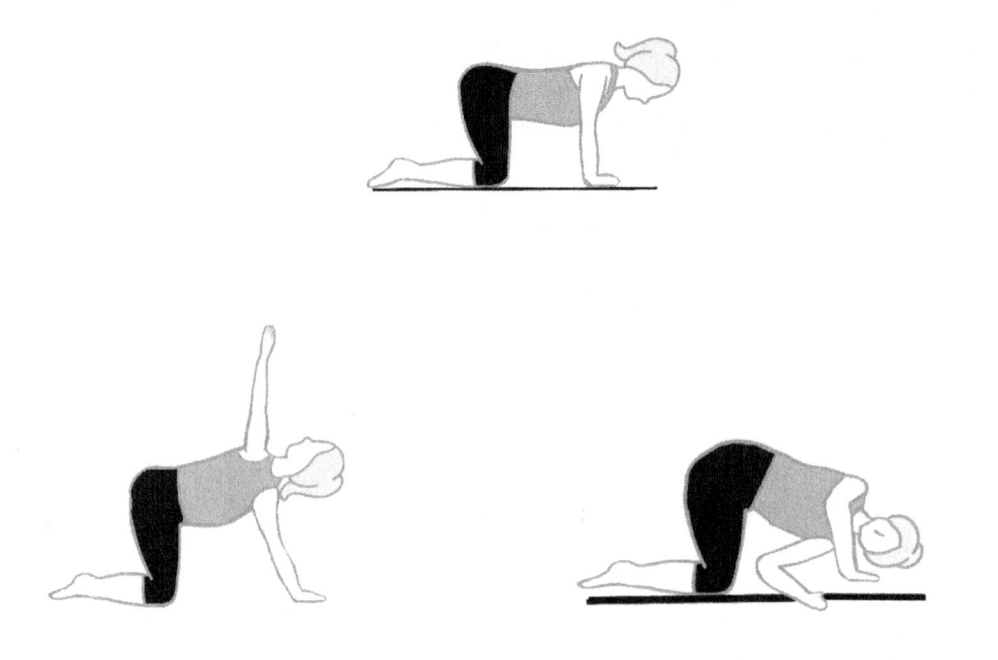

Cobra Dance Pose

- From table pose slowly stretch your legs back and lay prone.
- Put your hands underneath your shoulders with fingertips spaced forward.
- From here you' re going to arch gently your back lower, pushing down your hips, your palms, and the tops of your feet against the ground down. Lift your chest off the ground. Take a long breath to the rest the chest.
- Raise the whole torso, with arms outstretched and knees bent. Arch your torso up, with the head in your arms, to make the cat pose. Repeat slowly 6 times, trying to pace the breath.

Fish Pose

- Take the Tadasana pose on rug: supine resting position with face up relaxed, feet and arms fall open.

- Place a pillow behind you, under your shoulder blades.

- You will feel your neck, upper chest, and shoulders stretch. Hold fish pose resting on a pillow while you take about 3 breaths.

- Release and repeat holding the pose for 3 breaths.

- If it hurts to do this, relax and sit down. Listen to the sound of your body stretching and smile as the energy flows through your body.

Puppy Pose with Wall Pose

To practice additional stretching, do this exercise with your hands on the wall, about the distance of a chair.
Start from the Tadasana pose and, after a few breaths, kneel in facing the wall, using a blanket for better comfort. From there:

- Take a breath. Put your hands on the wall.

- Breathe out and push your chest and head towards the wall.

- Inhale. Move your fingers upward, along the wall.

- Breathe out and push your belly in and your hips out.

- Breathe in/breathe out. You will hold a puppy pose with your hands on the wall for approximately 6 breaths.

- Breathe in and relax your body.

- Breathe out and extend the stretch into the arms, deeper into the belly.

- Take a breath. Release the hands from the wall.

- Release the air, come and sit in the Vajra Sitting posture. This involves bending the knees backwards with the soles of the feet facing upwards and the big toes touching.

- If it feels good and comfortable, do it again.

- It's okay to support your knee with a blanket.

This is a good posture for stretching the chest and can be practiced at home 2-3 times a day without hyperextending the neck.

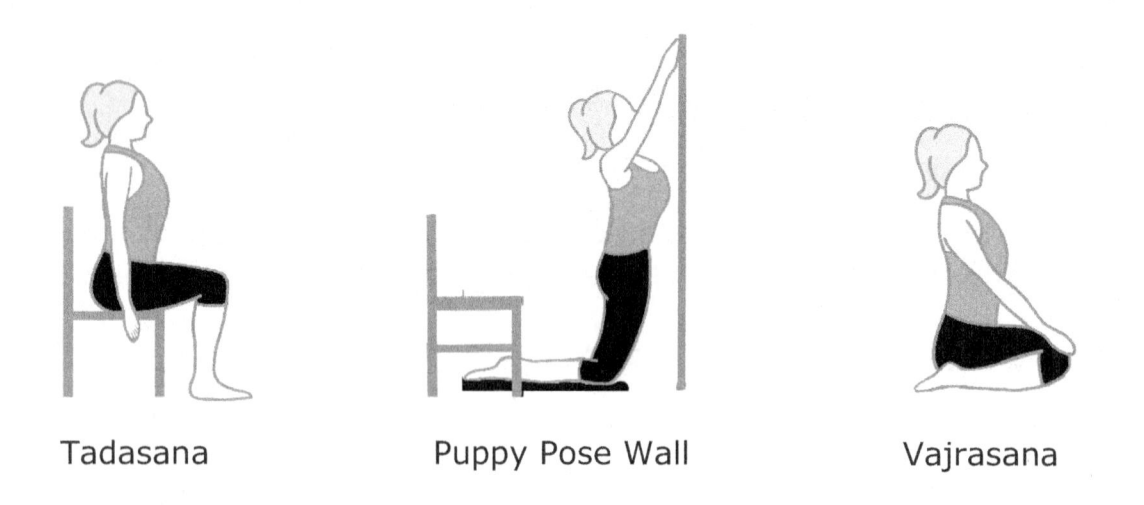

Tadasana   Puppy Pose Wall   Vajrasana

Circle of Joy Pose

- Relax and sit down. After a few rounds of breathing, start practicing pranayama while moving your shoulders, arms, and neck.

- This exercise is a great way to control your breathing while working your upper body.

- Move your arms in a circular motion for 3 rounds, which takes about 2 minutes. Focus on moving to the rhythm of your breath.

- The happy circle pose will help open your diaphragm muscles and help with the flow of your breath, thus releasing tension around the arms and shoulders. For comfort, it is recommended that you sit on a yoga mat.

Square Breathing

- It is always good to maintain peace of mind and body to enjoy yoga's benefits, so practicing pranayama as part of a yoga sequence is highly recommended.

- If you practice it, the mind becomes more focused, encouraging a full, deep, and smooth energy flow into the body.

- Similarly, sit on chair in Sukhasana posture: a relaxed posture with legs crossed, hands on knees and arms loose.

- Exhale gently through your mouth and inhale through your nose, hold your breath in each step, counting 4 seconds for each sequence.

Downward Facing Dog Pose

Chair steps with knee bending, this is a variation of downward facing dog:

- You will continue standing in front of the chair: take a breath, hold the chair, and move your feet back.

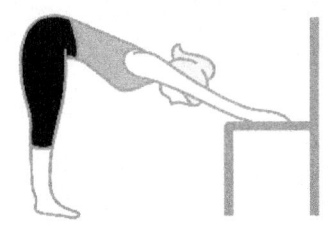

- Release the air: lean forward, extending the spine and flexing the hips.

- Inhale/exhale. Adjust the distance and hold in a downward-facing dog position. Bend your knees slightly.

- Inhale/exhale and hold this position for 3 breaths.

- Inhale/exhale twice and relax.

- Inhale/exhale. Hold the position again for 3 breaths.

- Proceed to bend your knees forward with the support of a chair so that you calm the stiffness of the hips in the lower spine. To improve blood circulation, stay parallel to the floor while extending the spine. Make sure the distance between you and the chair is comfortable.

Warrior Chair Pose

Here are the step-by-step instructions for practicing the Chair Warrior Pose

- First, have a chair handy. Chairs should be according to how tall you are. When seated, your feet should touch the floor. In this case, use a chair that does not have armrests.

- Start by aligning yourself with the Mountain Chair Pose. Sit on the edge of the chair. Stay there for 2–3 breaths.

- Take a breath and separate your feet. Start on the left side first. Open your left leg to the left, as in Chair Goddess pose, legs apart, and place the arms down (note: left leg only). Bring your knees in line with your ankles and hips creating a 90-degree angle.

- Hold your feet flat on the floor, toes facing to the left. The left thigh must rest on the chair.

- Release the air, straighten your right leg back, and straighten it at the knee. Here, the right foot should be flat on the floor with the toes facing forward. The Goddess Pose is about keeping the abdomen contracted and the back straight without curving it.

- Place your hands on your knees and keep your back straight. Sit nice and straight. Once your body is comfortable, take a breath and extend your arms to shoulder level. Make sure your palms are facing down, and your bows are not bent.

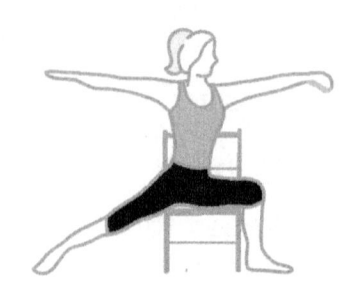

- To finish, turn your head and observe the fingers of your left hand. Confirm that your spine is straight and that your chest and shoulders are open.

- While doing so, ensure that your leg alignment has not changed and that your front knee is not bent to either side. Stay balanced on the chair for about six breaths. Proceed to breathe slowly, deeply, and gently.

- When you release, let the air go and turn your head toward the center. Lower your hands and align them back with your legs on the mountain chair. Stay like this for a while. Then follow the instructions above and do the stretch on the other side (right side).

- This time, you will open the right leg to the right, creating a 90-degree angle. Stretch your left leg backward, toes going forwards. Then, take a breath and open your arms at shoulder level, palms down. Finally, turn your head to the right to face your right toes while sitting upright with your spine straight. Stay like this for six breaths. Then release the air and return to the starting position.

- To finish, relax in the chair for 3 breaths.

Corpse Pose

Two variations of Corpse Pose with chair can be done.

The first is simply from a sitting position, comfortable, with arms and hands relaxed on the legs and legs stretched out placing a Bolster (or similar) under the ankles.

The goal is to look for a comfortable, supported and as symmetrical position as possible, to breathe slowly to concentrate and fully experience this moment of relaxation.

The other variant start from a supine position on a carpet, using a chair. Here are the steps for you to change from Corpse Pose to Chair Pose:

- Start by having a chair, yoga mat, and towels on hand. Place the mat on the floor and place a medium-height chair on top of the mat so that you get your upper body aligned with the rest of the mat. You should have a seat approximately 15–16 inches off the floor.

Fold the towel and place it on the chair for the comfort of your calves.

- Lie on your back on the mat with your hips close to the legs of the chair (not too close), bend your knees, and place your feet on the floor. To begin, carefully align the back of your upper body with the floor, with your arms slightly away from your body. Your palms should face the ceiling. When you widen the mat, be careful to rest your shoulders on it without pressing or straining them. With this pose, you will relax your neck, head, and jaw, and your forehead and face will be free of pressure.

- Now lift your feet off the floor and put your legs on the chair. Spread your feet hip-width apart. If necessary, realign yourself so that your knees and the back of your shin rest on the chair. Feel your lower backdrop to the mat and lift your legs up and down in the chair. Breathe naturally, watching the movement of your abdomen. Relax and close your eyes. Allow your upper body to sink into the mat, with your spine in its natural position due to gravity. Let the pose connect you to Mother Earth.

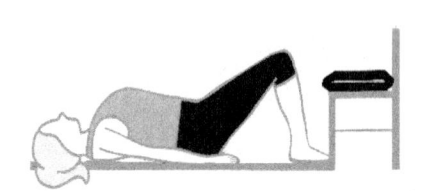

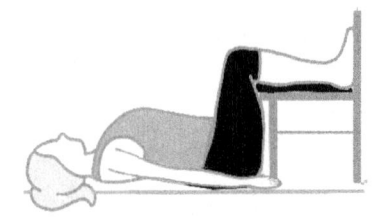

- You can do this for at least 5–10 minutes or as long as possible. Then, to release yourself from this position, start by lifting your legs off the chair. Bend your legs and bring them to your upper body. Twist the body to the right or the left. Stay like this and sit down. You can also do Savasana (corpse pose) after practice if you like.

Note: The sandbag method is suitable for people with weak feet. You can put a sandbag over your calf to stabilize your leg. Older people who have trouble lying on a mat or breathing difficulty can skip this exercise.

Chapter 6: Friendly Poses

This is a series of friendly poses that you are sure to love and that bring your body into harmony.

Connecting in Awareness

- Sit in a chair (a comfortable chair that allows your feet to rest firmly on the floor) with your knees together, feet together, chest out, shoulders back, and chin slightly up and straight.

- Start with normal breathing for about 3 or 4 repetitions. Then, when the breathing is smooth, and you are conscious, begin to breathe slowly and deeply. Place one hand on your stomach and chest and feel your body move with your breath. Expand the abdomen as you inhale and contract it as you exhale.

- See how the breath becomes deeper and softer as you inhale. Notice how the breath feels at the tip of the nose and how it moves down the back of the throat and into the chest.

- You will continue with this breath approximately 12 or more times while confirming that your body is relaxed and even, smiling as you do so.

Giving Love to Shoulders and Arms

The following chair yoga postures are performed in succession, coordinating the breathing process of each movement.

This flow is done about four times; you go deeper with each inhalation and exhalation.

The Flow

- Inhale through your nose and raise arms, sideways at shoulder height.
- Release the air through your mouth and entwine the arms in front of you.

- Take a breath through your nose and bring your arms straight up over your head.
- Blow through your mouth and bring your arms back down to your sides.
- Repeat 4 times

Mountain Pose Standing With Raised Hands

- In the mountain pose, take a breath and raise your arms so that the palms of your hands are facing inward.
- Proceed to stretch the arms and feel the stretch in the upper shoulders, neck, and upper back.

Hand Stretch on the Chair Top

- In the flow, exhale and stretch your arms up with fingers interlocked and palms facing up.
- Proceed to stretch when you feel the tension in the shoulders, upper back, and chest.

Seated Cactus

- Begin by inhaling and lowering your arms to shoulder level while seated.
- You will have your upper arms parallel to the floor and your forearms perpendicular to your upper arms as if forming an imaginary cactus.
- Breathe in and feel your shoulder blades, chest, and arms stretch as you feel your arms become stronger and tighter.
- Keep them aligned with the shoulders and chest as you get the chest to feel strong, confident, and relaxed.

Kundalini Circle

While sitting in a mountain chair:

- Take a deep breath: place your hands on your knees and lift your spine.
- Exhale and calm down.

- Take a deep breath: begin to move your torso to the left, then your face to the left of your hips.

- Exhale. Move to the left towards the left knee (if possible).

- Take a deep breath and move to the center, then to the right.

- Exhale and lift the torso from the right side.

- Inhale/exhale: move your torso in circles around while sitting in the chair, taking about four breaths.

- Inhale/exhale and repeat this movement counterclockwise for four breaths.

- Inhale, relax, and return to the mountain pose.

- This will help you release any tension around the abdomen, lower back, pelvic region, upper back, and neck. Sometimes just having the tension in your hips and shoulders can cause other bodily discomforts.

- As long as you stay in this position, make sure that the connection with the body and the breathing process is happening all the time. As in the case of most yoga postures, breathing is itself the healing process.

- This pose is an excellent way to recharge your body when the dynamic is over. As you do this flow, bring your attention to the base of your spine and tailbone, and connect with this stretch while keeping your body relaxed.

Twists Sitting on a Chair

- Relax and sit comfortably while doing a few rounds of breathing. Then turn on the right and place your right hand on the recliner and the other hand on your left thigh.

- Take a breath and slowly turn to the right, rotate your torso from the hips backward, and release completely.

- You will hold this seated twist while taking 6 breaths. With each exhale, twist further back and feel the stretch in the neck, upper back, abdomen, lower back, and buttocks. Return to the starting position calmly and relax.

- Take a breath and now repeat with the left side. Hold the position while taking 6 breaths. Release and relax as you return to the starting position.

- These types of twisting poses are always beneficial for better energy flow, as they strengthen and stimulate the organs while also reducing blocked ducts, stimulating detoxification, and, most importantly, releasing tension at the base of the spine. When the channels of Qi flow are unobstructed, the normal functioning of all body systems is stimulated.

- Proper functioning of the body's systems helps keep immune levels safe and under control.

To Open your Back

Following Yoga postures are performed in flows that are always good as they bring balance and stability to the body and breath.

The Flow on the chair

- Take a breath, raise your arms up in the chair.

- Release the air while you are in that position.

- Breath in, place your hands on your knees and take the Cat Pose. Exhale softly.

- Breathe in, raise your head, carry out a Cow Pose and exhale.

- Breathe in and raise your arms in the hands-up chair. Release the air while holding the pose.

- Take a breath, bring your hands behind your body and then assume the Cobra Pose, arching the chest forward and lifting the head.

- Breathe out, place your hands on top of your knees and relax.

- Starting with inspiration, repeat the three positions 4 times. Take a look at the following pictures.

CAT >   COW >   COBRA

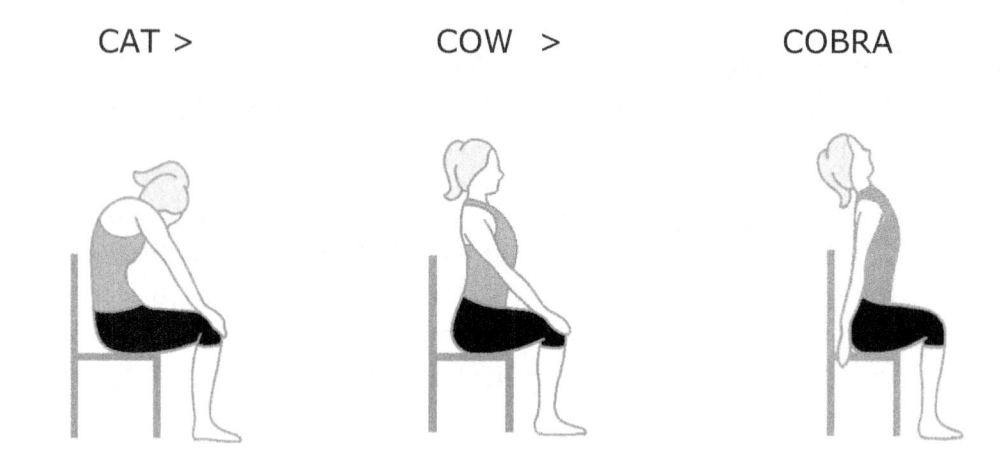

Raising Hands

- In mountain pose, take a breath and raise your arms above your head, open your chest, and fully extend your shoulders and arms.

- Raise your arms above the level of your heart, as this helps it to work properly. Gentle aerobic exercise is key to energizing the entire body and stimulating the nervous system.

This pose helps relieve stiffness from long hours of sitting. It is a great way for you to stimulate your chest and heart while connecting with your breath.

The Seated Cobra

- Inhale deeply and raise your hands by holding on to the back of the chair.

- Do gentle backward bends that will help relieve stiffness in your neck, shoulders, and back.

Pigeon on the Chair

- Sit in a mountain pose and do a few rounds of breathing.

- Start by taking a breath. Place your right foot on your left knee while bending at the hip.

- Release the air: when you feel the stretch at the top of your hamstring and inner thigh, push your right thigh down with your right hand.

- Feel the stretch all the way down.

- Inhale/exhale: calm down and lie on your back in mountain pose.

- Breathe in: place your left foot on your right knee.

- Inhale/exhale: hold the position for 6 breaths as you sit up straight and extend the spine.

This is a great way to relieve lower back stiffness by focusing on stretching the hamstrings and glutes. When you feel stiffness in your lower back from sitting for hours at a time, you can relieve this by stretching the leg muscles, in this case, the hamstrings and glutes (hips).

Upward Facing Dog

- Start from the Tadasana pose standing in front of a chair.

- Take a breath and stretch your arms up.

- Release the air, approach the chair, stretch your arms, and rest them on the seat. Step back to lengthen your body, with your legs parallel.
- Breathe. Push your arms up, to lift your chest and shoulders, looking straight ahead.
- Exhale. You are in Upward Dog.
- Inhale/exhale to balance and lengthen your legs, shoulders, chest, and arms as you push up, with your hands firmly on the chair

- Inhale/exhale, hold the position while taking about 6 breaths; take a breath to deepen the back bend.

- Inhale/exhale, release, and stand in Tadasana pose facing the chair.

Backbends are a great way to open tight muscles in the lower back while encouraging deep breathing. Proper breathing is important to keep the nervous system, and other body systems stimulated and healthy.

Table Pose Raised to Gain Stability

This pose is done in front of a chair:

- Take a breath while resting your hands on the chair.
- Release the air, stretch your arms, bend your head and neck.
- Inhale: Bring your right leg behind you and extend your foot as far as possible while holding on to a chair for support.
- Breathe out, and bring your right knee forward as you bend.
- Inhale and straighten your leg back again.
- Inhale/exhale and hold the position while taking about 6 breaths; hold the legs straight in the tabletop position while standing.
- Inhale/exhale: stretch your hips and legs back as you look down or up.
- Inhale/exhale. Then release and relax back into the Tadasana pose.
- Inhale/exhale and now do the same with your left leg, keeping it straight behind you for 6 breaths, bending your right knee forward over the chair and head down.
- Inhale/exhale. Then release and return to the Tadasana pose.
- The standing table pose is also done with the chair and can be done alternately with each leg or holding each position for about 6 breaths.

Extending your legs back is a great way to open up your lower back muscles and will help with flexibility and hip stability. All of this will serve to get you at a desk for long periods without feeling tired or heavy at the end of the day.

It's a great way for you to move your hips by making your lower body strong (mainly your legs and glutes). It helps to improve balance and make your leg muscles strong and your body balance as you work both sides of your body.

High Lunge Pose

- Stand in front of a chair.
- Take a breath and lift your left leg over the chair.

- Release the air and propel your torso and hips forward.
- Breathe in while keeping your body relaxed.
- Release the air as you push your torso forward at rest. Place your hands on your waist.
- Inhale/exhale as you do the high lunge pose with the chair, ensuring your feet are firmly planted on the floor and the chair.
- Inhale/exhale holding the position for 6 breaths as you push your hips and torso forward.
- Inhale/exhale as you release and relax back into the Tadasana pose.

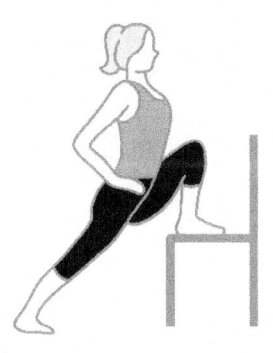

- Inhale/exhale now repeating the movements with the other leg, pulling the left leg back while pushing the right leg into a lunge.
- Inhale/exhale holding the position for 6 breaths.
- Stretch to open the leg muscles while reducing tension in the lower back, hips, and psoas muscles.

Triangle Pose

- Sit towards the edge of the chair, in mountain pose.
- Inhale and extend the left leg out to about 90 degrees with the foot on the ground.
- Exhale as you place your right foot at an angle of about 45 degrees.

- Inhale as you lift your arms and twist slightly to the left.
- Exhale as you lower your left hand to the floor and lift your right arm.
- keeping the triangle pose.
- Inhale/exhale as you stretch your torso to the left and hold the position for about 6 breaths.
- Return to Mountain Pose to relax.
- Perform the same exercise on the opposite side synchronizing breathing.

This is an excellent pose to release tension in the lower and upper back while calming the psoas muscles that tend to accumulate stress in the body, including emotional stress.

This pose is also like a gentle opener for the heart, which helps you to have deep, easy breathing.

Reverse Warrior Pose

This exercise resumes the "Warrior pose", with one more movement.

- Let go and sit in the chair. Take a few breaths with your back straight and lengthen your spine.
- Then relax into the Mountain Chair Pose.
- Inhale, rotate the left leg to the left and rest the left thigh on the chair.
- Exhale and extend your right knee and right foot out to the side.
- Inhale and move the right leg slightly to the right, with the foot on the ground. As you inhale, bring your arms up as well.
- Breathe out and slide the right hand down the right leg, bowing the body to the back and looking up at the left arm that follows the torso.
- Breathe and straighten the body and return to the starting position to relax.
- Start over with the opposite side. Left leg extended to the left (foot out to the side) and right leg to the right bent at 90 degrees with the thigh on the chair.

- Follow with arms to do reverse warrior pose.
- Take 6 slow, deep breaths on each side.

To close, get back the position of the mountain and relax.

Gentle backbends are a great way to open up the hips while helping to bring energy into your body. Feel both sides stretch evenly as you breathe slowly and deeply to maintain balance.

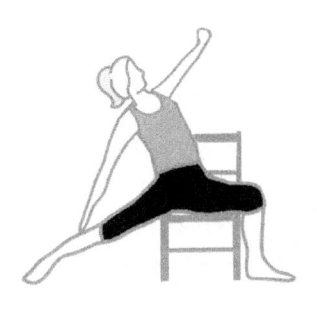

Chair Boat

You're going to use a chair to put resistance into the movement, and it's a creative way to make it easy and fun.

- Sit in the chair.
- Inhale and bring your legs up while holding them with your hands as in the chair pose.
- Exhale and bend your knees while moving your legs and ankles, if necessary.
- Inhale and squeeze the buttocks and legs.
- Exhale and stretch your back and legs. Use your core muscles to balance your legs.
- Inhale/exhale and hold the position as represented in the drawing.

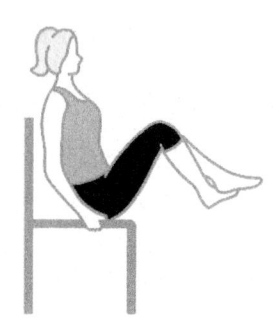

- Inhale/exhale and now contract your quadriceps, abdominal muscles, chest, shoulders, and pelvic muscles; you should maintain balance for about 6 breaths.

- Inhale/exhale as you lower your legs and relax into the mountain pose.

- Repeat all the movements.

This pose is a great way to exercise the trunk and abdominals to help keep the body and mind strong and alert, respectively.

It also serves to generate energy in the body after long hours at a desk.

Pose Upward Straddling

- Sit in Mountain pose to restart.

- Extend your legs out in front of you and, if possible, straighten your knees.

- Open your hips and extend your legs.

- Sit upright, extending your arms, shoulders, and chest.

- Elevate your legs as high as you can with your right arms. The purpose is to get your toes as near to your hand as possible.

- Hold the stretched position for a couple second.

- Now relax to sit in comfortable pose.

- Repeat if you like, balancing the breath during each step.

With this pose, the core muscles, hip openers, leg muscles, biceps, and triceps work hard, and the pelvic floor muscles gain strength. Everyone strikes a great pose (you don't have to be in a full pose), so you develop strength, stability, and overall body endurance.

Wind Release Pose

- From the chair, start with the mountain pose.
- Inhale and bring your legs up, placing your feet on the chair.
- Exhale. Now bring your knees to your chest while holding them with your hands.
- Inhale and relax your body.
- Exhale. Pull knees inward; sit up straight.
- Inhale/exhale releasing all the air.
- Inhale/exhale. Sit up straight with your thighs pressed together as you exhale and hold the position for approximately 6 to 12 breaths.
- Inhale, release, and relax into mountain pose.

This is a great way to relax the lower back, shoulders, and arms. It also serves to calm the digestive system, which can become sluggish after prolonged sitting at a desk.

Downward-Facing Dog in a Chair With Knees Bent

- Sit in a chair in the mountain pose.
- Inhale and stretch your arms, then place them on the chair.
- Exhale, bend your torso, and extend your arms, shoulders, back, and hips. At the same time, keep your knees bent if necessary.
- Inhale/exhale while keeping the posture down and bending your knees.
- Inhale/exhale. Hold the stretch with each exhale; take about 6 breaths.
- Inhale/exhale. Release tension and relax.

Bend the hips and torso forward to relieve lower back and shoulder stiffness. This pose also helps with the flow of oxygen and blood to the head, which further serves relaxation and leaves space for clear thinking.

Standing Squat Pose

- Inhale facing the chair (resting your elbows on the chair or on the top of it).
- Move your hips out and extend your arms (elbows on the chair).
- Exhale, bend your knees and pull your stomach in.
- Inhale and relax your body while toning your feet, hips, and shoulders.
- Exhale and squat down.
- Inhale/exhale. Stay in the standing squat pose with arms crossed in front of the chest.
- Inhale/exhale. Hold the chair for about 6 breaths.
- Inhale, stand up, and release.
- Inhale/exhale: repeat the standing squat position, arms crossed in front of the chest, and hold for 6 breaths.
- Inhale. Release pressure and relax into a mountain pose.

Squats are a great way to open up the hips and get you to pay attention to your body and its extension. It helps the hips, knees, lower back, and quads, as these are the areas most affected when you have to spend a lot of time sitting.

Forward Fold with Two Chairs

- Sit on one chair, stretch forward your spine and arms then relax for a few laps as your breath becomes softer and slower.
- Next use the second chair, in front of you to support the bust, head and arms even with the use of a cushion, for complete relaxation.
- Breathe for about 24 repetitions, watching the movement of the abdomen and chest.

With each breath, you will explore your whole body, starting to relax from the tips of your toes to the top of your head and then from the tips of your toes to the back of your neck.

Variation

- You can put your legs on another chair and stretch your back and legs doing the Savasana pose.

- Keep your breathing relaxed.

- Relax and hold the pose for 24 breaths or about 10 minutes.

- You can finish the sequence by chanting OM... 12 times, then rub your hands together to complete the sequence.

Half Seated Pose

- Sit in the middle of the chair with hands on seat, extend your right leg and place your right foot on top of your heel.

- Raise your toes and press firmly on your heels; stretch the soles of your feet. Connect with that stretch and hold for about 6 breaths.

- Now gently lean your torso forward, stretch your quads, hamstrings, calves, and the soles of your feet, for 6 breaths. Let yourself go and relax.

- Now repeat the movements with the other leg; try to hold the leg harder for a longer time. Repeat this stretch as much as you can.

- Sitting in a semi-inclined chair is a good way for you to work the tendons and tissues near the plantar fascia (ligament).

- Release and sit with your feet in your sleep.

Leg Lift Pose

- Sit in a chair and do not lean your back against the backrest.

- Straight back, breathe easily, and sit comfortably with your feet firmly planted on the floor. Never rest only your toes; try to keep your feet flat on the floor.

- Bring the foot forward with the heel on the ground and lift your right leg up, parallel to the floor. Keep your toes straight and your leg as straight as possible.

- Hold the position by squeezing the knees and quads. Keep your breathing coordinated by doing approximately 6 repetitions while lifting one leg.

- Release and repeat with the other leg.

- The key to this exercise is that you feel the stretch in your ankles, soles, and calves. What you will do is gradually open the soles of your feet, and in the meantime, the other muscles do the stretch with your feet over your knees and hamstrings, so you keep the soles of your feet healthy.

- Let yourself go and relax

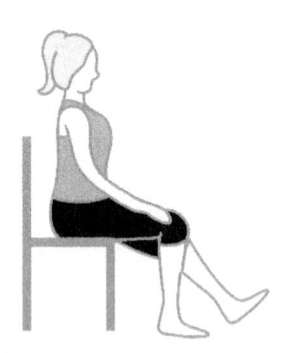

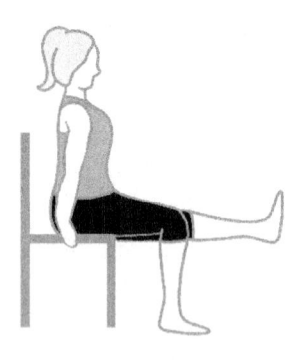

First Step   **Second Step**

Stretched Side Angle

- Sit on a chair. Inhale and place your left thigh sideways on top of the chair. Exhale and straighten your right leg to where your knee and ankle stretch.

- Inhale. Put your right arm on top of your head.

- Exhale and bring the left forearm over the left thigh. Take a deep breath, tilting the body to the left, pushing with the right arm, beside the head, looking up. Take 3 breaths.

- Come back to standing position and switch to the other side, laying the right thigh on the chair

- Now repeat and hold this position for about 3 breaths. Inhale/exhale, release, and relax completely.

Lateral trunk flexion is done while stretching the hamstrings and lower back which serves to generate energy in the body.

This posture also serves to open the vitality channels, allowing prana to flow easily. Prana is important, as being healthy means being harmonious in mind and body.
The motto is Keep them calm and cool.

Gently stretching to the side while keeping the lower body centered will serve to understand the awareness of stretching better. Understanding stretching will help facilitate your healing process.

In this posture, the buttocks are stretched, as well as the lower and middle back, hamstrings, and inner thighs.

Conclusion

By now, you know that yoga makes your body more flexible and helps you cope even with medical conditions. When we stretch and lengthen our muscles, we increase our ability to move them and improve their elasticity and the tissues connected to them. This strengthens posture, reduces injuries, or relieves injuries you may have, not to mention it feels good.

While greater flexibility is one of the most well-known benefits of yoga, we can't forget about strength. However, with regular practice, you can find significant increases in core muscle and endurance. This has many advantages for those who cannot participate in more traditional forms of exercise.

Yoga Improves Balance and Coordination

With yoga, you are required to use your body in other, more challenging ways. This can help improve balance, coordination, and proprioception (the ability to sense where your body is in space). When you improve these skills, you can reduce the risk of falls and injuries.

Your Mind and Body Become Better Connected

One of the unique features of yoga is that it requires you to have full attention to the present moment. This can help improve the connection between your body and mind and your body awareness and movements. Regular practice will teach you to control your body with greater precision and ease.

Your Circulation Improves

By practicing yoga, you help your organs pump oxygen-rich blood throughout your body, including your organs and tissues. This can lead to better overall health and function. In addition, improved circulation can help reduce pain and inflammation.

Your Posture Improves

When you lengthen and stretch your muscles, you can stand better and move more easily. This helps reduce pain and stiffness and improves overall appearance.

Lower Your Stress and Anxiety Levels

Not surprisingly, one of the main benefits of yoga is that it reduces stress and anxiety levels. This practice helps you calm and relax your mind and body, which leads to a decrease in stress hormones such as cortisol. In addition, yoga helps you increase serotonin and gamma-aminobutyric acid (GABA) levels, which are known to promote relaxation and calmness. This will also help with your sleep habits.

As a final reminder, keep in mind that each of the yoga poses should be done with careful attention to each step. If you feel it hurts, stop; if the intuition, the muscle, that part of your body says no, it's no. It's okay to push it a little bit to do the job, but do not overdo it because you could end up with serious consequences, an injury, or if you exercise to alleviate a problem, you can aggravate it even more.

Printed in Great Britain
by Amazon